THE WAY OF HERBS

The Way

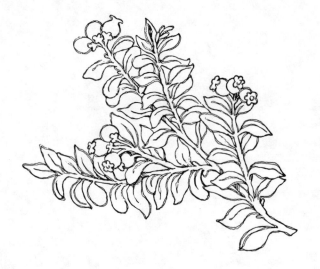

Edited and supplemented by
Subhuti Dharmananda, Ph.D.

UNITY PRESS

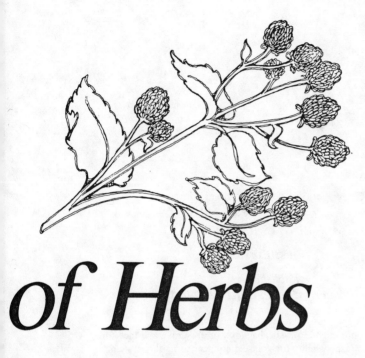

# of Herbs

by Michael Tierra, C.A., N.D.

Illustrated by Robin Spowart

SANTA CRUZ

Library of Congress Cataloging Data

Tierra, Michael, 1939-
    The way of herbs.
    Bibliography: p.
    Includes index.
    1. Herbs — Therapeutic use.   I. Title. [DNLM: 1. Herbalism — Popular
works.   2. Herbs — Popular works.
WB925 T564w]
RM666.H33T53   615'.321   80-12190
ISBN 0-913300-43-8 (pbk.)

Typeset in Times Roman by Jonathan Peck
Cover Design by Bill Prochnow

PRINTED IN THE UNITED STATES OF AMERICA
135798642

Dedicated to my teachers: Dr. Christopher, Hari Das Baba, Foon Lee Wong, Miriam Lee, Efrem Korngold.

TABLE OF CONTENTS

provided. Both the common and botanical names are listed along with the part of the plant most frequently used, the systems of the body affected by the herb, the essential properties and methods of preparation, with special attention to dosage.

Factors affecting the potency of herbs are discussed. Included are the species of plant used, the method of preserving it, the storage conditions and the duration of storage. This information will help you decide which herbs are best and in which form to purchase them.

Following a few simple rules, you can combine herbs into effective formulas that will prove superior to using the herbs individually. In addition to the "primary" medicine, "secondary" medicines, including stimulants, antispasmodics and demulcents, are used to balance the herbal effects. Two dozen valuable herb formulas are provided, including tonics for the liver and kidneys, an eyewash, a heartburn formula and a healing salve.

Internal and external treatments for a wide variety of ailments are given, with formulas, dosage information and notes on maximizing the effectiveness of the treatment. Includes such topics as arthritis, cramps, fevers, hemorrhoids, poison oak, vaginitis and weight reduction.

Herbs are safe and without side effects when used properly. However, one must have adequate knowledge of the potential hazards of herb use. Among the important concerns are the irritating effects of essential oils, the problem of overdose and cumulative effects, cautions concerning the use of herbs in pregnancy and for children, the FDA evaluation of herbs and the need for proper consultation with trained healers.

LIST OF ILLUSTRATIONS

EDITOR'S PREFACE

Michael Tierra has been practicing herbal medicine and acupuncture in Santa Cruz, California for the past decade. He has an extensive background of study with traditional healers of America, India and China. From these diverse cultures, he has developed a unique approach to herbalism that is firmly rooted in practical experience. I have also been deeply involved in herbal medicine, but with a background in biochemistry, physiology and practical pharmacology. Much of my work has been with investigations of herb safety and efficacy from a scientific viewpoint. For years, Michael and I have been working and teaching in Santa Cruz, representing two very diverse aspects of herbal medicine. In that time, I have come to gain a deep respect for the traditional medical systems that gave rise to much of our current knowledge and Michael has gained a keen interest in the scientific explanations and clinical evaluations of herb action. It was therefore most appropriate and timely that we should join forces in producing this book. From the original manuscript Michael provided, we have developed a valuable synthesis of the many aspects of herbal knowledge that make up "The Way of Herbs."

I am often asked the question: "Do herbs really work?" I answer both yes and no. The human race has been practicing medicine for many thousands of years and from all available reports, it has been reasonably successful. Herbal medicines have been a large part of all medical systems over the millenia, but they have been put to a very hard test by the severe conditions of a developing world. The greatest assault on health has come from the unsanitary conditions of city life and from bad diet. The unequal distribution of foods leaves some individuals without adequate nutrients while giving others deadly dietary excesses, especially in the form of highly processed foods. Where practiced, improved sanitation and proper diet have done more for health than any medicine that has ever been used. Few people seem to manage these conditions in their lives, and so medicines are required to perform a monumental task.

Herbal medicines have worked very well for those who have used them properly, and the literature is replete with success stories. Many remedies have been consistently recommended across cultures and time on the strength of their efficacy. In fact, most modern pharmaceuticals are based on chemical constituents that were at one time isolated from the traditionally used herbs (although a large number are now being derived from bacteria, fungi and animal sources as well). So I must say that herbs work.

Modern pharmaceuticals are directed against symptoms. They act swiftly and powerfully to remove the symptoms of disease. Compared to this type of action, it would seem that most of the herbs do not work. For in many cases, an herbal treatment will be gentler and more gradual in its action and it will rely primarily on allowing the body to heal itself by a slow, natural process. Using herbal therapy, the body will become stronger and the individual will take the time to learn something about the factors that led to the disease in the first place, thus giving the opportunity to prevent reoccurrence. The quick and powerful action of modern pharmaceuticals will bring superficial relief. Their primary action is to give temporary relief from the responsibility of taking proper care of one's health. These drugs, when relied on in this way, will lead to a more severe disease later. For you will have only pushed aside the warning signals that you are doing something wrong. Herbs don't work that way.

However, too many people turning to alternative medicine try to cure themselves by using "a sprinkle of herbs in a cup of boiling water," thus drinking what they think of as an herbal tea. This will accomplish nothing. It is a great myth that drinking beverage teas will cure ailments and provide a healthy life. It is one thing to eliminate the bad habit of drinking coffee and black tea by replacing it with an herbal beverage, and another thing to treat an ailment with a potent medicinal tea or other herbal therapy. Herbal therapies will generally require a fairly large dose of herbs and an extended period of treatment. In fact, it is important to continue the treatment beyond the point where the symptoms have vanished, to bring strength to the deepest levels from which the ailment had sprung forth.

Many of the mild herbs need to be taken in the amount of one ounce per pint (two cups) of water in making a tea. This will yield about one and one-half cups of tea, which is to be taken a half cup each time, three times daily. Other herbs, with stronger action, are taken as alcohol extracts (tinctures) that are about four times as concentrated as a tea, or in capsules that are sometimes taken as frequently as every two hours, two capsules each time (sixteen per day). The herb tea bags found in a store will usually have only about one-fourteenth of an ounce of herbs; the bottles of prefilled capsules will often have the instructions "take one or two capsules daily." These instructions are generally not for therapeutic use of the herbs. (Small "homeopathic" doses are valuable only when the proper formulation is applied according to the principles of that medical system.) When treating acute diseases, the therapy will be applied for several days, and chronic ailments may be treated over a period of months.

It is not possible to overemphasize the value of a dietary change in treating an illness. It will be difficult to obtain success with herbal therapy or any therapy without proper attention to the role of diet. It is very important that upon becoming sick, one immediately eliminate hard-to-digest foods, using a simple but nutritious and balanced diet. Then the energy that goes to digesting foods and dealing with toxins in the diet is no longer diverted from the essential process of healing. Once the crisis of the acute ailment is over, it is necessary to progress through dietary changes to correct the imbalance that allowed the illness to appear and to strengthen the body against further disease.

In his practice, Michael gives considerable attention to the condition of the patient in terms of the Oriental concept of balance between Yin and Yang, and he has made extensive notes on the subject. Here, however, we have attempted to present this valuable aspect of diagnosis and treatment in a way easily accessible to our Western readers. The concept of Yin/Yang balance suggests a basis for many healthful dietary changes, as well as for determining the best herbal therapy. It is a major point of departure from the modern Western approach to health and disease. Michael also relies heavily on the use of Ayurvedic diagnosis and treatment, but this field of study is still quite difficult to present in a book such as this, so most of the references to these techniques have been reserved for a subsequent work. There both the Chinese and the Ayurvedic systems will be presented, and adequate space devoted to full explanations of both theory and practice. These traditional methods do not replace, but augment, modern medical diagnostic practices.

In the "Kitchen Medicines" and "Herbs to Know" chapters we have tried to eliminate any information that would not be of immediate use to the reader. Those who wish more information may consult the sources described in the Bibliography. We have provided dosages and descriptions of methods of application, and the number of herbs has been restricted so as to minimize the common problem of information overload found in many herb books.

The chapter on "Obtaining and Storing Herbs" is based on my own experience, not only as an herbalist, but as a person who has worked with herb companies that produced the herb products you find in retail stores. I suggest that the reader take special note of the concern for the species of the plants and also the form in which they are purchased and stored.

If you will observe carefully the rules for "Making an Herbal Formula," you will find it easy to produce a very large number of useful and effective herbal preparations. The formulas presented are those that Michael feels are among his most valuable, and most of these clearly fit the general formulation technique. A few are less obviously derived from the rules set down, but they are nonetheless useful recipes and indicators of the range of herbal preparations. Some modifications have been made to allow the formulas to be produced from herbs available in stores or by mail order. If you are able to gather fresh herbs, these can be used and many substitutions can be made, so that local herbs will be generally adequate for the entire formula.

I have also added the chapter titled "Cautionary Notes on Herb Use." It will be important to read this section carefully and observe warnings presented there. I have done considerable research into the problems of herbal toxicology, but this field is poorly developed. The majority of concerns have briefly been presented in this chapter.

I am often asked if herbs are safe. To this, I again answer both yes and no. When herbs are used properly they are as safe as any natural food and they are far safer than other drugs. When used improperly, they can cause a number of unpleasant effects, and can even cause death. While there are many mild herbs that need to be used in fairly large doses, there are also some very potent herbs that must be used in relatively small doses. Herbs should not be used without an adequate knowledge of their traditional uses and application. When the body reacts negatively to any therapy, it is important to look carefully at the dose, and the appropriateness of the treatment. We have placed a number of cautionary notes throughout the text. When herbs are used properly, they are not only safe, but they are without side effects.

In collaborating with Michael in producing this book, I have taken special care to include much practical information for one not only to get started using herbs, but even to proceed towards the point of becoming an herbalist. You will find information here that has not

been collected into any other single reference source. On the strength
of this knowledge, you can move to familiarity with other herbs and
techniques as necessary.

I have long been interested in providing an accessible education in
herbal knowledge. Working with the Herb Trade Association and
Dr. Paul Lee of the Academy of Herbal Medicine, I helped produce
three major Symposia on herbs, which brought together university
researchers, government officials, herb suppliers and herb users. The
Symposia have led to an ongoing interaction between such groups
to bring out the important knowledge of herbs from many vantage
points. The Third International Symposium on Herbs eventually led
to the establishment of the Institute for Traditional Medicine and
Preventive Health Care. Established in 1979, the Institute carries on
research and education with emphasis on herbal medicine. An advisory
board of cooperating scientists from around the world has assisted
our organization in its efforts. Active coordination of international
research projects is a major part of the emphasis of the Institute.
Projects underway include: evaluation of ginseng in the prevention
of heart disease; prevention and treatment of ailments of the female
reproductive system; study of tobacco substitutes and herbs that can
be smoked to alleviate the symptoms of asthma and bronchitis; the
use of herbs with disinfectant, antiseptic and antibiotic activity. The
Institute also has an agricultural research station in the Catskills,
Cold Mountain Farm, where it is evaluating methods of production for
a variety of important medicinal herbs, including American ginseng,
goldenseal and lady's slipper.

Two research associates with the Institute are Calvin Cohen and
Grace Marroquin. They have helped extensively with the preparation
of this book by reviewing all the sections, making numerous valuable
comments and suggestions and providing helpful insights. Both Grace
and Cal have contributed their own herbal knowledge as well as experience in apprenticeship with Michael and myself. They are currently
involved in carrying out clinical trials of herbal treatments.

Among our tasks in studying herbs has been the review of the
literature to separate out vital information from that which is frivo-
lous or outright incorrect. We have come to consider *The Way of
Herbs* a unique book about herbs. Unlike most other herbals, it
restricts its references to just over a hundred herbs, concentrating on
important medicines that can be used again and again in a wide variety
of treatments. The information about the herbs has been centered
around the nature of the systems affected and the important properties of the herbs. Other aspects of the herbs, such as their history in
medicine, growing region, appearance and minor uses can all be

learned from the other books mentioned in the Bibliography. We have deliberately focused on ways you yourself can learn to use the herbs.

I have included a few herbs in the "Herbs to Know" chapter that I have studied and used, but that Michael has not generally prescribed. These include kava kava, stoneroot and tienchi, herbs that are subjects of our research projects. In addition, I have provided a section on smoking herbs in the "Methods of Application" chapter. This is a method that Michael also uses, but it is of particular interest to me in terms of our research regarding asthma and bronchitis. As a result of Michael's very high regard for echinacea, which we hope has been adequately brought out in this book, our research group is in turn undertaking a detailed study of this herb as an antibiotic and blood purifier.

Rarely does an herb book provide any insight into the proper method of formulation and preparation of herbal therapies. *The Way of Herbs* provides the basic information necessary to use not only the herbs presented, but also any other herbs, in both the formulas presented and in formulas that you will design to fit your basic needs. This book contains the most comprehensive guide to date to the potential problems of herb use, from inadequate concern for the diet, to insufficient dosage, to excessive use. In addition, this book contains the most detailed instructions yet available for the methods of herbal application, both for the therapeutic techniques and for the production of useful herbal preparations in your home.

It has been very difficult to obtain good information on Chinese herbs despite the fact that their use is becoming very popular. From the thousands of herbs available in Chinatowns, Michael has picked the most widely used and highly valued to introduce to our readers. The herbs are well worth the trouble to track down and purchase, for they are superior tonics among the range of herbs available. This is the only book that details the use of these herbs in a context that the Western reader can readily understand.

The Way of Herbs thus brings together the most important aspects of several herbal traditions. It will be an invaluable contribution to every library of herb books and an essential manual for all who wish to practice herbal medicine effectively.

SUBHUTI DHARMANANDA, PH.D.
*Institute for Traditional Medicine
and Preventive Health Care*

*Santa Cruz, California
June 1980*

INTRODUCTION

The Herbalist's Path

It is a mistake to view herbology only as a science studying the therapeutic properties of plants. More than this, the path of the herbalist is a cultivated attitude towards nature and all of creation. I remember the time that I spent with the Karok Indians of northern California— whenever I presented one of them with an unfamiliar plant, the inevitable question was "What's it good for?" Certainly the Indians love nature as their home, but rather than merely holding an aesthetic viewpoint about it they combine a sincere appreciation for its beauty with a functional attitude based on the idea of "use, not abuse." This is also the attitude of the herbalist towards nature. It is in contrast to the lack of appreciation demonstrated by those who retreat to the wilderness to dump all of their repressed desires symbolized by the beer cans, pop bottles and other debris left in their wake. The view of the herbalist is also in contrast to the many pseudo-ecologists who make futile attempts to maintain natural environments as aesthetic monuments with no functional purpose, leaving signs saying "do not touch," "do not pick the plants," etc.

The herbalist, along with the American Indian, appreciates nature not only for its beauty but also for the valuable resource of wild foods and medicines that grow in these all-giving bowers. Thus the herbalist views nature as a positive force, and as a provider and teacher. Everything is seen as having a purpose that can only be revealed if we learn to be patient, and engage our senses both subtle and gross in allowing us to trust and understand the secrets this teacher can reveal. Nature communicates her secrets directly to us in terms of forms, colors, fragrances, sounds and flavors as well as by way of the more subtle information that comes to us through our intuitive imagination.

A certain perspective is necessary for this communication to occur. We must cultivate an attitude of respect for all living plants and animals and accept them as a gift. We must learn not to slight even the smallest living thing, while maintaining an attitude of deep reverence and gratitude. This will enable us to better understand what benefit we can be for each other's evolution. The way of the native Americans shows us a reciprocity, a give-and-take attitude about nature. In northern California no real cultivation of food was done; everything was found and gathered in the wilds. However, the forests were periodically burned to keep down the underbrush, keeping the ground clear for gathering acorns, dynamizing the soil with fire and ash, encouraging the growth of edible herbs and berries.

At first when we enter into an unfamiliar natural sanctuary, we may only recognize one or two familiar plants. Rather than ignoring them or taking them too lightly, we should see them as friends and diving messengers whose presence may allow us a welcome security and familiarity until we learn about the many other unfamiliar plant-friends growing in the area. Everything has a purpose and a use because everything has qualities and properties. It is part of the human's divine purpose to become more conscious and aware of the environment we all share.

While it may be our ultimate destiny to transcend nature, we must first rediscover our rightful place in it. Those of us who have grown up in cities have of necessity suffered from a separation from nature. I remember living in a wilderness community during the late 1960's. During the first few months, I mistakenly attempted to come to terms with my relationship to the strange yet exotically attractive forest where I lived by doing the only thing my previous conditioning would let me conceive of—going out each day with my rifle in hand and playing the role of the great white hunter. Thankfully I was so inept that any halfway intelligent animal could hear or sense my approach from a long distance, and I never bagged anything during that period. It was during those days that, perhaps partially out of embarrassment from coming back each day with nothing in hand, I became attracted to the wild herbs of the forest and each day brought back various specimens to identify.

At this time we harbored a number of black beret revolutionaries who were seeking temporary refuge from the confusing and paranoid vibes pervading cities and ghettoes. They evidently felt threatened by the strangely peaceful forest, with its gentle quiet streams and new fallen snow. Somehow they became very frightened of the raw quiet and deep silence. They often imagined some terrifying animal, a projection of their inner distrust and unfamiliarity with the environment, uneasily expecting something to issue forth from that profound natural peace and eat them alive—or perhaps some governmental authority might be hiding behind a big Douglas fir tree, just waiting to get them. In any case, no matter where they went, it was an absurd picture seeing them strutting in their most downtown "macho" attitude, wearing their black beret and always carrying a pistol or a rifle. This was the only model they had for dealing with the unfamiliar.

It seems that after a while, when people realize that they are alone and nothing will eat them, they begin the often destructive process of letting down their societal inhibitions; then we find the tendency of country folk to spend their free time drinking, getting high and ultimately making themselves sick. Through such ignorance we miss the incredible lesson that nature has to teach us, the lesson of how to just *be*. Nothing to compete with (except perhaps the squirrels for the spring harvest of hazelnuts), no egoistic posturing for a job or a raise, no struggle with the Russians for the oil of the Middle East, no desperate search for approval or acceptance from societal peers or acquaintances. Nature offers us a rare freedom from the painful and stressful concerns of society.

The path of the herbalist is one path that can offer a vital link to the natural and interaction with nature's wilds. It gives us a point of view by which we can see ourselves as being connected with the entire process of life. It has been stated that in very ancient times everyone was born with knowledge of the use of herbs. Eventually, some of that was lost due to the development of extended societies leading to the development of future civilizations. During that transitional period people began to look to the wild animals and birds to guide them in understanding the healing power of herbs and plants. The American Indian, for instance, would watch the bear, who was considered to be the closest, physiologically, to the human, and learn what it would eat both for food and for medicine. Ayurvedic medicine has many herbs named after certain animals, such as one called garuda bhuti, named after an eagle—probably because it was first found in eagles' nests. The Chinese still use precious nests of certain birds in a soup considered to be of great benefit as a whole-body tonic.

While such indications are often valuable, it was discovered that there were exceptions. One hermit yogi sadhu, for example, would eat only those foods that he saw monkeys eat. But one day he was discovered poisoned and dead because he had eaten one thing which, while not poisonous to monkeys, proved to be a deadly poison to humans. For this reason, certain principles, ideas and concepts had to be extracted from our previous experience with natural foods and medicines in order to safeguard and deepen our understanding. Humans began to observe more closely the various colors, shapes, fragrances and tastes, along with the geographical location and season in relation to the healing and nutritional properties of plants. It was from these beginnings that the study of herbology evolved.

The first thing to emerge in the classification of herbs was a recognition of their cooling or heating properties. Thus it was noted that everything was encompassed by a cycle of polarity of night and day, sun and moon, wet and dry, male and female, hot and cold, full and empty, light and heavy, smooth and rough, etc. It was further observed that there was in fact a relationship between these obvious characteristic qualities and certain disease conditions of the body. An individual with a hot disease such as a high fever was treated with a cooling, detoxifying medicine such as a cool fruit or the tender leaves or petals of a flower such as hibiscus, elder, yarrow, red clover blossoms, mint, etc. Diseases characterized by coldness, weak digestion, poor circulation, etc., would be treated with deep rooted herbs and plants or barks of certain trees that would affect the deeper organs and secretions of the body, such as ginseng, dandelion, prickly ash bark, bayberry bark, burdock root, etc.

As ancient as this discovery was, this basic hot and cold relationship of plants and diseases is still a fundamental principle of all natural healing. Of course, there is much more to it than this, and as with any complex system, it is made complex by superimposing one clear and simple thing upon another over and over until it seems to defy our total comprehension. Thus the path of the herbalist may also encompass the laboratory with the identification and extraction of certain vital biochemical agents found in herbs.

There is an ever increasing danger of becoming far too out of touch with nature—not only external nature but, perhaps, our internal psychological nature as well. The herbalist must cultivate an attitude to maintain his or her balanced connection with the vital roots of existence. Such ritual practices as talking or praying to a plant, making an offering before picking or harvesting it or bringing the first-picked herbs to the people who live in that area will help to raise and maintain one's consciousness at a level necessary for the proper practice of herbal healing. It must be understood that herbal healing involves a specially directed and trained imaginative and intuitive sense that cannot be taught mechanically but must rather be discovered and acquired with practice.

True "holistic" healing involves a healing of both mind and soul, and native shamans, curanderos and medicine men and women are always very aware of this fact. Using various tricks and performances to entice and help others to see themselves in a more positive way, they offer herbs as plant-sacraments providing a specific point of focus for all of their creative play. The herbs became what the Hindus called yantras or sacred objects, gross (more perceptible) manifestations of subtle healing energies.

The herbalist's perspective remains with him or her wherever he or she may travel. I often wondered how I would fare as an herbalist if I found myself in a foreign country where I could not identify a single plant. I almost found myself in such a place when I lived for a few weeks in a village in southern India. I barely recognized one herb, except gota kola, which grew everywhere as a common weed. Yet within two weeks, with a little personal effort (such as checking a few botanical books on the area but, most important, asking questions of the local folk), I learned the medicinal use of several plants, enough to prescribe them to the villagers for their various ills. They appreciated this for the same reasons as people everywhere appreciate being reminded of those simple and valuable things that can be found growing freely around them such as the common weeds.

In walking through wilderness trails and discovering wild plants and herbs, one should take the opportunity to notice the many conditions under which herbs and plants grow. An herb growing in one locale may be better suited for particular diseases than one growing under a different set of climatic conditions. For instance, we can find chaparral growing in veritable stands and fields in high desert places throughout the western United States. Recently I discovered a few chaparral plants growing on a high windy peak in Baja California under conditions quite different from any of the other chaparral I had ever previously gathered. Upon tasting a leaf of this specimen, I noted it was much less bitter than the common desert chaparral. Just as the climate and outward conditions of our life affect our characteristics and personality, so also do the growing conditions of a specific area affect the characteristics of the medicinal plants that can be found growing there. I decided that this particular "Baja" chaparral was especially good for diseases involving the liver because of the traditional relationship in Chinese medicine between the wind and the liver.

Other considerations I have noted for various reasons are as follows:

1. Herbs growing on the north side of a mountain are more tonifying and strengthening because of the increased power and stamina they must develop in order to survive in a more difficult growing area.

2. Herbs growing in lowlands or near water are more beneficial for urinary diseases.
3. Herbs growing in high, dry desert regions tend to be of more benefit to the spleen and pancreas because they would help the traditional function of the spleen-pancreas according to Chinese medicine, to transform moisture in the body.
4. Herbs growing in fertile, nitrogenous soil would be of more benefit for the digestion and assimilation. Also herbs whose job it is to fix nitrogen in the soil, including the leguminous plants such as clover and alfalfa, would help in our metabolism of proteins and cell formation.
5. Herbs growing in cold, harsh weather tend to be more building and heating in contrast to herbs growing in hotter, more temperate climates, which would tend to be more eliminating. While both can be detoxifying in their respective ways, there is a subtle but important tendency manifested by herbs found growing in different geographical localities.
6. The tastes of herbs are important indicators of their properties. The sweet taste is nutritive; pungent is dispersing; salty taste influences water balance and digestion; sour is digestive and cooling; bitter is cooling and detoxifying. Many herbs have a number of tastes and therefore a number of properties.
7. As we walk, often a plant will greet us with a striking scent. It is a known fact that the sense of smell has a direct connection with the subconscious mind. It is one of the powers of aromatic herbs and plants to help us to get more consciously in touch with our subconscious process. Aromatic herbs such as mugwort, pennyroyal, bay, sandalwood, rose, sage, etc., can be used in special talismans and dream pillows to help the individual get more in touch with their dreams and psychological processes. Usually these aromatic herbs can be used internally in a variety of ways, ranging from a sweating tea in fevers (the volatile oils of aromatic plants are eliminated through the pores of the skin), to antibiotic treatment of internal infections of the bladder, lungs, etc., to digestive, carminative herbs for better assimilation.

When you are gathering herbs, take time, make your peace with the environment and its life as well as with the living plants that pass their life cycle there. Avoid the tendency to plunder and pluck about unconsciously. Before taking an herb, offer a prayer of thanksgiving or a good thought of appreciation. Herbs have feelings not at all dissimilar in many respects to our own, and we and they can both be persuaded to give more of ourselves and our energy if we can be genuinely persuaded to feel good about the process. In any case, never take more than a third of the foliage of a plant. Never strip the bark around the entire circumference of a tree unless you deliberately intend to kill it. Bits and pieces can be taken from various parts of one tree and from various trees, and each tree can still heal itself over.

During various seasons, the vital energy of herb plants is found in different parts. In the spring it is in the newly formed leaves and buds; in the summer it is in the fruit and blossoms; in the fall and winter it is in the roots. These are the best times for gathering these various parts of medicinal herbs and plants. If there is only one or two specimens don't bother them. Always gather where there is an abundance — then you can be certain that the herbs you get are potent. When drying the herbs, carefully spread them out on a screen in a well-ventilated, partially shaded place. Turn them once each day so they will dry evenly, thus preventing decay and browning of the leaves.

In conclusion, we might direct our attention not only to the powerful beneficial aspects of medicinal plants, but also to their ability to poison and inflict harm. Poisonous herbs are used in minute "homeopathic" dosage, often one part in thousands, to effect profound cures of both acute and chronic illnesses. In any case, never eat a strange herb or plant of which you have no positive identification. There are methods of determining whether certain herbs are poisonous or not but all of these involve tasting them, and there is some question whether this is 100% effective; there is thus always the chance that you could have an unfavorable reaction.

The path of the herbalist is to open ourselves to nature in an innocent and pure way. She in turn will open her bounty and reward us with her many valuable secrets. May the earth bless you.

THE WAY OF HERBS

1

BALANCE: THE KEY TO HEALTH

A Deeper Understanding of Health and Disease

Health is a reflection of the balance between the different aspects of ourselves (body, mind, soul) and our environment, our experiences, our associations and our food. There cannot be sickness in any of these categories without its being reflected to some degree in all of the others.

The cornerstone of all natural healing is summarized in the statement *"all healing comes from within and the body heals itself."* Before any true healing, as opposed to mere symptomatic relief, can occur, two important prerequisites must be met:

1. understanding the basic cause of our sickness on all levels, physical, emotional and spiritual;
2. being willing to surrender to our own deepest wisdom and implement whatever positive alternatives may appear to be helpful.

It is a mistake to reach for a remedy before taking the time to acknowledge the two foregoing conditions. Strong allopathic drugs with dangerous side effects may give quick symptomatic relief but are often the cause of weakness and diseases that may occur later. Even natural remedies such as herbs, vitamins and dietary changes may be inappropriate if they are not accompanied by a good healing attitude. We will develop a healthy attitude when we finally choose to see our problems from a larger perspective, as a process of readjustment or as valuable lessons to be learned.

I believe that there is an eternal force that drives us onward through countless changes, trials and errors. As a stream must follow its long course through the forest and mountains, flowing sometimes gently and smoothly while at other times encountering obstacles and rapids, so our life must flow through its various changes. We cannot hold ourselves back from experiencing those changes. *Such opposition is the primary cause of all sickness.*

The incessant yearning for an ideal may be said to propel us through these changes, including changes of health and disease. In this sense there are no accidents. Rather, we are moved by the silent force of evolution, which, more often than we suspect, foils our most careful plans and our expectations of staying the same. Life has evolved in adaptation to an ever-changing environment. As it attains the blossom of consciousness, it develops within each one of us the capacity to generate the changes and the lessons that will effect yet a higher adaptation and awareness.

It is essential to realize that every disease has a positive aspect. The ailment informs us of our resistance and of our imbalance and it provides a focal point for discovering all the negative energies we have cultivated. In the healing process, our lessons are learned and the body is brought naturally back to a reflection of total balance. If we fail to see the positive aspect of a disease, it will not be possible to get rid of the negative aspects.

We put ourselves in situations that cause illness, and thus create our sicknesses, for several reasons:

1. to grow and learn;
2. to help foster compassion in ourselves and others;
3. to repay old "karmic" debts that we may be carrying;
4. to provide an excuse for death to occur;
5. to get love and attention.

None of these reasons involves such matters as bad diet, accidents or self-neglect—all the usual diatribe offered in most well-intentioned discourses on natural healing. *The fact is that bad diet, accidents, self-neglect and other "causative factors" are themselves a reflection of the sickness we are experiencing.* They, along with the physical symptoms that must ultimately follow, are also only symptoms rather than the deep underlying causes.

A disease healed naturally leaves a person stronger. In the natural process of healing we come to understand our weaknesses and thus replace them with true strength. The highest form of ancient healing made no attempt to cure disease but rather sought to sustain the individual through the use of mild foods, herbs and spiritual disciplines as the individual healed himself, from within and completely, body, mind and soul. Any attempt to offer a remedy that would stop the natural process from occurring was considered an interference with the integrity of the individual's own self-generated healing process. As Lao Tzu put it in the *Tao Te Ching*, "A person will get well when he is tired of being sick."

The knowledge and the use of certain herbs and foods was a prerequisite among the ancient healers. Herbs, unlike the synthetic chemicals of most modern medicines, promote the natural functions of the body. They play an important part in the process of strengthening from within. Yet they are effective only if the other manifestations of the disease are also corrected, especially the diet. Enduring changes in the lifestyle, intended to remove unhealthy dietary practices and unnecessary stress, can only be made with the proper spiritual realization. Thus any treatment of an illness must take into account the needed spiritual growth of the individual. Disease gives us the opportunity to reach a higher consciousness. The process of healing is a reflection of our new awakening.

2

THEORY OF USING HERBS

The use of herbs can be a very simple healing art. In fact, it has long been known as the "Art of Simpling." Herbs were known as "simples" because a single herb could be used to treat a wide variety of maladies. I once helped a woman on a Canadian Indian reserve gather red alder bark, of which she would make large amounts of tea to drink instead of water. The tea cured her of her lower back pains and of a problem of frequent urination; it also helped normalize her blood pressure. On another occasion, I was preparing a tea of freshly picked mugwort and comfrey to be used as a wash to relieve someone's poison oak. This same herbal brew was subsequently used for someone who had a sprained ankle; on another who got a deep scratch from a frightened cat; and finally, for an individual who was suffering from a bad case of indigestion and who got relief by taking a few teaspoons of the tea. Sometimes older people and others suffering many sicknesses and feeling very weak come to me and say, "What herb should I take?" My favorite reply is "Any herb."

If one goes to the bookstore and looks through herb guides, it is not uncommon to come across encyclopedic works with the complexity of hundreds of herbs used in numerous special formulas. Herein lies a danger to anyone practicing herbalism: getting lost in this complexity and being separated from the basic and simple experience of involvement with a few herbs. There is, of course, a place for this complexity, for ultimately the complexity of the herbs must match the complexity of the individual. However, everyone can begin with the most important principles of Simpling.

THREE PRINCIPLES OF SIMPLING

The first principle is to use the herbs that grow nearby. The type of illness that is contracted in a particular area is somewhat dependent on the environmental conditions. For example, prople in northern climates tend to suffer conditions of bronchitis, while people in southern climates tend to suffer from parasitic infections. Similarly, the herbs that grow in that area take on the characteristics of their environment and are particularly useful for the treatment of those ailments associated with the climate and other conditions of the area. In any region, there are perhaps a dozen important herbs that can be used to treat most illnesses encountered there.

The second principle is the use of mild herbs. Mild herbs can be taken freely and will exert a general effect on all the body systems, aiding in the process of healing many different types of affliction. Thus almost any herb of mild action that grows in the area may be used.

The third principle is that these mild herbs must be used in large doses. Since the herb is very mild, only in a large dose will it have the power to overcome most illnesses.

Perhaps the most important lesson I have learned in my training as an herbalist has been to use large doses of these mild herbs. There is an important difference between beverage teas, which use only a small amount of the herb, and medicinal teas, which use much larger amounts. Too many people are drinking herb teas to cure their ailments thinking that a sprinkle of herbs in a cup of boiling water will do the trick. In general this is not the case. One may need to drink several cups of a much stronger tea for several days to effect a satisfactory cure.

ADDING COMPLEXITY

The local herbs will effect a cure when properly used over an extended period of time by bringing the healing energy of the environment to the user. For a quicker change in one's condition, it may be necessary to reach out to other places to find herbs useful for this purpose.

The complexity of herb use comes when a person is:
1. unwilling to use the large doses of mild herbs;
2. impatient for relief of symptoms;
3. eating a diet derived primarily from foods of other climates, foods eaten out of season or processed foods;
4. unwilling to devote the time and energy to identify and gather the local herbs.

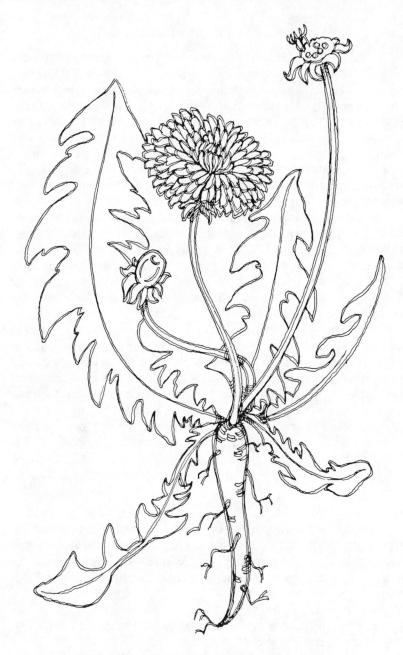

DANDELION (*Taraxacum officinale*)

*A nutritive herb that clears obstructions
and stimulates the liver to detoxify poisons.*

Unfortunately, most of us fit one or more of the above categories. In such cases, one must become familiar with a much larger variety of herbs and must be careful in adjusting the dose to account for their powerful effects. The herbs will be used in basic formulas that complement and balance their properties to make them applicable to the specific ailment and constitution of the user.

No matter which approach one uses, in order for an herbal treatment to be truly effective it is essential that the individual eliminate the factors causing the illness. The components of the lifestyle, especially the diet, have the greatest effect on the balance of the body.

DURATION OF TREATMENT

In general, for most acute ailments one will obtain favorable effects in just three days by using herbs and making the appropriate adjustments in the diet and other components of the lifestyle. Even so, one should continue the herbal therapy for one to two weeks after the symptoms are gone to insure a more complete healing and avoid reoccurrence of the ailment. Because the herbs have a beneficial and normalizing effect on the whole body, other physical conditions, which were not the main object of the therapy, will also be improved. If a positive experience from the therapy has not been obtained within about three days, it is necessary to change the herbs being used.

Herbs are also used in the treatment of chronic diseases of long standing. In this case, several herbs are compounded together into a balanced formula to be taken over a period of time at the rate of two or three cups of tea a day. It is important to understand that these chronic diseases have been developing over a long period of time and have probably involved a number of organic functions as well as a major adjustment on the emotional level. For these reasons, one may not get immediate results, although occasionally someone will report significant improvement even after only one week. One can generally expect to require about one month of treatment for every year the disease has been developing.

If one is undergoing such an extended period of herbal therapy, it must be understood that the body, as with everything else in nature, functions cyclically. That is, there is a period of maximum effectiveness in the use of herbs, and that effectiveness is benefited by regular breaks in the program. I adopt the "cycle of seven" as a standard. Of the seven days in each week, one day should regularly be reserved to fast and forgo the taking of herbs, thus giving the body a rest and preparing it to respond with renewed vigor after the fast.

The main problems that arise in the use of herbs are lack of commitment, lack of consistency, insufficient or extreme dosage, a formula that is not specific enough and last, but perhaps most important, a wrong diet.

THREE FUNCTIONS OF HERBS

One must be able to coordinate the various herbal qualities as closely as possible with the nature of the individual being treated. Herbs have three general functions in the body and are compounded according to the state of the individual. The three functions are:

1. eliminating and detoxifying—using eliminative herbs that act as laxatives, diuretics, diaphoretics and blood purifiers (see the chapters on "Herbal Therapies" and "Herbal Properties" for definitions of these terms);
2. maintaining—using herbs that counteract the physical symptoms, allowing the body to heal itself;
3. building—using herbs that tone the organs.

The first stage in an herbal treatment is generally to eliminate, removing toxins that are both a physical cause and a result of the disease. However, this step causes some depletion of energy and should not be used for persons who are weak or who are suffering a long-term degenerative condition. Instead, one uses herbs to build up the system for those who are weak, such as those recuperating from disease, and those with recurring sickness. Whether eliminating or building, an herb that stimulates the overall process is included in the formula.

For persons suffering long-term degenerative diseases or very severe symptoms of an acute disease, the first step is to use herbs that will maintain the body through the crisis and stabilize the condition. Once this has been achieved, it is possible to proceed with the appropriate use of elimination and building.

Persons who have a diet rich in animal products and refined foods have a special need to eliminate toxins and have a characteristic condition for which leaf and flower herbs are most effective. Others who go to the opposite extreme and have a diet rich in raw vegetables and fruits also need to eliminate toxins, as they usually suffer from poor assimilation, and are best treated by the roots and barks of the herb plants (see the chapter on "Diagnosis and Treatment").

Herbs can also be regarded as special foods and it is often of great benefit to take several herbal tonics to aid the major systems of the body. For convenience these are taken in pill or powder form or as a tincture (see the chapter on "Methods of Application"). These tonics bolster the organs of the body and are useful in preventive medicine as well as in the treatment of chronic diseases and congenital weakness. One may, for example, simultaneously take a kidney tonic, blood purifier, lower bowel tonic, glandular balance formula and an herb tea that is specific for a particular ailment. Such a combination may be taken in full doses of each tonic separately, or the formulas may be combined to form a single dose made up of smaller amounts of each component. The former is a full-potency treatment, while the latter is a maintenance dose that is usually satisfactory for long-term treatment and prevention. In this way, one may begin to match the complexity of the individual with a complex herbal program.

3

HERBAL THERAPIES

There are a number of ways in which the body responds to herbal treatments, and these have traditionally been divided up to produce a basis for eight general methods of therapy. These methods are:

1. stimulation;
2. tranquilization;
3. blood purification;
4. tonification;
5. diuresis (control of fluid balance);
6. sweating;
7. emesis (vomiting);
8. purging.

Each therapeutic method is suitable for particular kinds of diseases, and it is often appropriate to combine several methods for the most effective treatment.

In applying therapy of any kind, one must regulate the treatment according to the energy of the body. Thus while the use of certain herbs to eliminate toxins through purging or emesis can be very effective, they are not appropriate for one who is weak or of low energy since these methods will reduce the body energy further. *It is important, then, to follow the changing course of the disease each day and to decide which therapy is most appropriate for that condition.* Familiarity with these eight therapeutic methods will make it possible to choose an effective course of treatment to promote quick recovery.

STIMULATION

The purpose of this therapeutic approach is to stimulate the vitality of the body to throw off the sickness. Herbal stimulants, when combined with other herbs, will promote their functions of eliminating, maintaining or building. Effective herbal stimulants include ginger, cayenne, garlic, black pepper and cloves. (A very useful stimulant formula, composition powder, is described in the chapter on "Making an Herbal Formula").

Stimulants increase the metabolism, drive the circulation, break up obstructions and warm the body. It is particularly useful to apply this therapy in the beginning acute stages of a disease. The body's underlying strength can then be stimulated to throw off the disease. The herbal stimulants can also restore vitality that has been reduced by chronic diseases.

Many ailments are attributable to blockages in the natural flow of blood, lymph, nutrients (digestion and assimilation), waste products (from food and metabolism) or nerve energy. Stimulants are an important means of breaking through these blockages, which are cold, inactive areas of the body. The increase in energy, circulation and warmth brings back the normal activity. Thus the dynamic balance of all aspects of the physiology may be restored.

Ailments characterized by reduced energy, causing one to feel slow and sluggish (as with colds and flus), are successfully treated by stimulant therapy, usually in combination with other therapies. In addition, prolonged, low-grade fevers may be treated with warming herbal stimulants such as black pepper and cayenne. In this paradoxical situation, the fever may be neutralized as the body is aided in its natural production of warmth, thus allowing the fever to subside.

Stimulants are also commonly used to overcome sluggish digestion. Many of the aromatic culinary herbs and spices are useful in treating indigestion and gas by stimulating the action of the stomach and small intestine.

Most people are familiar with the current campaign against the use of stimulants, particularly coffee and black tea. Despite the charges against the use of such beverages because of their stimulating properties (attributed to caffeine and related substances), the proper use of stimulant herbs is, according to herbal traditions, beneficial in treating a wide variety of conditions. The extensive use of stimulating beverages without regard to bodily needs will, on the other hand, be harmful. But most importantly, the major problem with coffee and, to a lesser extent, black tea is that they have a notable acidic effect, producing toxic conditions in the blood and digestive tract when taken in large amounts. This eventually contributes to the development of other ailments. Thus one should not confuse these overused beverage stimulants, which have a clearly detrimental effect, with other herbal stimulants, which, when properly administered, are very helpful in the treatment of certain diseases.

Stimulant therapy is not to be used when there is extreme weakness, as often occurs after severe and prolonged disease, since there is then no basic strength to stimulate to a better action. Stimulants, however, may be slowly added to help other herbs maintain the body through this critical time and build back the strength. Stimulants are also not used when the body is eliminating toxins through the skin in the form of eruptive skin diseases, since the use of stimulants will enhance that elimination process and make the disease symptoms appear worse. Minimize the use of stimulants in cases of nervousness and hypertension. Finally, stimulants, including hot, spicy foods, should be avoided when there is chronic imbalance in the colon. The stimulants will overwork this organ and may lead to problems with elimination and hemorrhoids.

TRANQUILIZATION

This therapy is used when there is great unrest, nervousness or irritation interfering with the process of overcoming the disease condition. There are three types of tranquilizers: demulcents, nervines and antispasmodics. These treatments may be taken intensively over a period of one or two days, as often as every hour.

Demulcent herbs and soothing foods will lubricate the joints, bones, gastrointestinal tract and even the irritating conflicts of our lives. Herbs such as slippery elm bark, marshmallow root and comfrey root, and foods such as warm milk and watery oat or barley cereals, are used to comfort and quiet a person while the process of healing carries on. Any mucilagenous substance will be effective; it may be taken along with warm milk and honey to promote its soothing effects.

Nervines are substances that feed the nervous system and balance its energy. These are also called nerve tonics. The nervine herbs include skullcap, catnip, wood betony, lady's slipper and valerian.

Antispasmodics calm the nervous tension in muscles, including both the skeletal muscles and the smooth muscles of internal organs. These also help relieve pain due to tension or convulsion. Herbal antispasmodics include lobelia, valerian, kava kava, black cohosh, and dong quai.

In all cases, it is important to have adequate calcium in the diet since this strongly affects the function of the nervous system and muscles.

It is not uncommon to use tranquilization therapy along with stimulant therapy. The tranquilizers will not counteract the stimulants, but will buffer their effects.

BLOOD PURIFICATION

Most herbalists agree that if one can purify the blood and neutralize excess acidity, all diseases will eventually subside. For this reason, blood purifiers occupy a prominent place in herbal therapies.

The blood and lymph of the body carry a variety of toxic substances, most of these being acids. These substances include constituents taken in with food and drink, such as chemical preservatives, which the body cannot easily eliminate. Also included are natural wastes of the body, which may be produced in excess, or inadequately eliminated, when the body's organs are functioning improperly. In traditional Chinese medicine theory, the toxins of the blood are considered excess "heat," and toxin-producing infections are called hot diseases. The site of the body most responsible for the purity of blood is the small intestine, which must separate useful nutrients from the totality of substances ingested. Secondary organs affecting blood purity include the liver, kidney and colon.

There are several ways to purify the blood:
1. directly neutralize acids with the strong alkalinizing effect of some herbs (e.g., dandelion and slippery elm);
2. stimulate the vital organic functions of the body, especially the liver and kidneys, lungs and colon (e.g., Oregon grape root, goldenseal);
3. dry excess moisture and remove excess fat where toxins are retained (e.g., plantain, mullein, chickweed, gota kola);
4. eliminate excess "heat," especially from the small intestine (e.g., rhubarb root).

The best herb for blood and lymph purification is *Echinacea angustifolium*, sometimes called "prairie doctor" or "Kansas snakeroot." It contributes to some extent to all these ways of purifying the blood. Other useful blood purifiers include: burdock root, dandelion, red clover, sarsaparilla, sassafras and Oregon grape root.

The use of blood purifiers is particularly important for the treatment of infections. Not only does the herb help remove toxins produced by the infection, but it can also remove the excess moisture that provides the medium in which it grows. Furthermore, the infection may be totally eradicated because the herb will stimulate our natural defense mechanisms. For example, echinacea promotes the production of white blood cells which can then destroy the invading bacteria or virus.

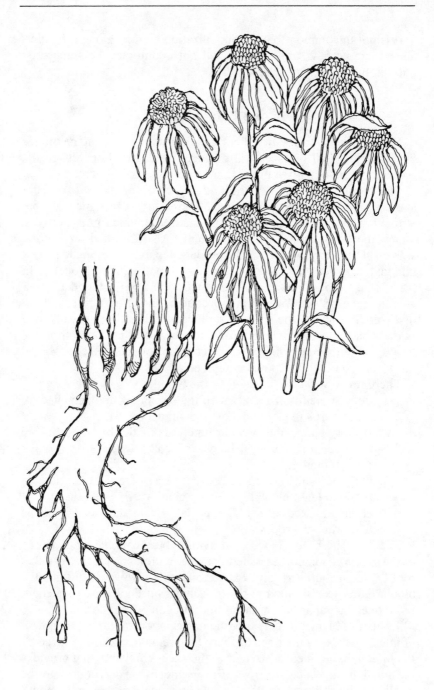

ECHINACEA (*Echinacea angustifolia*)

"King of the Blood Purifiers." A valuable alternative to antibiotics.

TONIFICATION

Herbs that can build the energy of the organ systems are used as tonics. They are commonly recommended for those who are weak and run down, having low vitality. Tonic therapy is used in the recovery from acute ailments and in building energy back for those suffering chronic diseases. It is also useful in maintaining a healthy condition and overcoming minor imbalances.

Tonics are nourishing to the organs. Some of the herbs act primarily to provide nutrients: vitamins, minerals and sugars. These are referred to as Yin tonics (see chapter on "Diagnosis and Treatment"), the most valuable being the seaweeds (kelp and Irish moss), alfalfa, comfrey and dandelion leaf. Others, in addition to providing some of these nutrients, act to balance and stimulate the energy of the organs, improving their ability to assimilate and utilize nutrients. These are the Yang tonics, the most valuable being the Chinese root tonic herbs (see chapter on "Herbs to Know"), burdock, dandelion, parsley, Oregon grape root and goldenseal root.

Tonic herbs are used to counteract a deficiency (weakness or critical shortage) in the body. Usually if the body is deficient in one function, there will be deficiencies in all the other functions and in the vital substances (minerals and vitamins). When one is very weak and out of balance, the use of strong, stimulating Yang tonics is not advised, as these will drive the system further out of balance. Therefore, the milder acting, nutritive Yin tonics are first used. These are usually the fruit, flower and leaf herbs. Later a stimulating tonic can be added to improve the assimilation and use of the nutrients. These Yang tonics are usually roots and barks.

The science and art of tonic therapy for treatment of chronic diseases, recovery from acute crisis and prevention of all ailments is most highly developed in the Far East. Several of the most important Chinese tonic herbs have been included in the chapter "Herbs to Know."

DIURESIS (CONTROL OF FLUID BALANCE)

The body fluids are comprised mostly of water. Through the control of this vital element, we are able to restore and maintain health and well-being.

The amount of fluids in the body can change very quickly. Our emotions are strongly linked to the balance of fluids in our bodies and thus can also change very quickly. In fact, changes of emotion are frequently related to changes in the water balance. For example, women commonly experience emotional sensitivity just before their menstrual period. At this time, these women are experiencing an increase in retention of body fluids. As the fluids are released during the period, the emotions again fluctuate and are eventually returned to the normal equilibrium.

Having too much water retained in the body leads to feelings of weakness, paranoia and depression. Too little water in the body, on the other hand, may result in explosive anger and other forceful reactions. Water may be used to quiet the "fire" but too much water will "dampen one's spirits." Excessive water, especially when taken in with meals, will disrupt normal digestion by diluting the stomach's acids and enzymes. The internal organs may also become waterlogged; a common example of this is the occasional occurrence of hypoglycemia due to a waterlogged pancreas.

The primary method of reducing water in the system is through the use of diuretic herbs. Important diuretic herbs include: prince's pine, buchu leaves, horsetail, cleavers, corn silk, uva ursi leaves and juniper berries. The use of these herbs increases the flow of urine, decreases the blood pressure and helps purify the blood. Diuretics are also useful for weight loss by removing excess water, and for this purpose it is good to use the astringent diuretics such as cleavers and uva ursi.

To maintain a good water balance in the body it is important to regulate the intake of water. When thirsty, check the cause of the sensation. If it is due to spicy foods, it may be necessary to reduce the amount of spices in the food so as to reduce the intake of water. On the other hand, if one is thirsty following exercise, the thirst is a natural response to water loss. A large amount of fluid is taken in the water content of food. Persons suffering from excess water in the system should switch to less watery foods. The amount of fluids taken in with foods should also be limited for all persons, since excess water will interfere with digestion.

When undertaking a program of herbal treatments, one may need to consider the amount of water taken as tea, and if this is too much, use other methods of preparation such as tinctures.

Kidney weakness is also treated by the use of diuretics. The weakened kidneys may be further burdened by excessive water intake. A clear physical sign of waterlogged kidneys is bagginess or darkness under the eyes.

SWEATING

Sweating is used to treat externally caused diseases such as cold, flu and fever. There are two methods of treatment: one with relaxing diaphoretic herb teas and the other with stimulating diaphoretic teas.

Relaxing teas, such as those made with catnip or lemon balm, are used to treat ailments where the pores of the skin are closed and the energy has retreated from the surface. The volatile oils in the herbs exit through the pores of the skin, soothing and calming the body surface. The stimulating herbs provide heat, increase the circulation and promote sweating. They are used to treat weakness in the internal organs. Useful stimulant diaphoretics include teas made from boneset, elder flowers and peppermint, or a combination of cayenne, ginger, lemon and honey.

The herbs used for sweating are taken as warm teas. The same herbs, taken as cool teas, are useful as diuretics. Sweating occurs to some extent just by taking the tea, but is promoted by providing additional external heat to the body, such as taking a hot bath and then covering up with blankets, after taking two cups of the hot tea.

EMESIS (VOMITING)

Emetic herbs induce vomiting and thus quickly empty the stomach of its contents. This may be a necessary treatment if one is feeling sick from eating too much food or a poor combination of foods. It is also recommended for treating poisoning by non-caustic substances that will not burn the esophagus when vomiting is induced.

Some people tend to create excess mucus as a result of certain foods they eat. The first line of treatment is to empty the stomach, where the mucus originates. Similarly, emetics can be used to treat colds that have resulted from overeating.

Ipecac, an herbal syrup found in most drugstores, is an excellent emetic. Lobelia can also be used. This is done by taking a full teaspoon of lobelia tincture (see chapter on "Methods of Application" for how to make a tincture) three times within an interval of about thirty minutes. In between taking teaspoons of lobelia tincture, one should drink as much peppermint tea as possible (about two quarts would be ideal) and tickle the back of the throat with the fingers to stimulate the emetic reaction.

Emesis greatly reduces the energy of the body and so should not be used by persons who are already very weak. The emetic treatment may be followed by a mild stimulating treatment, along with soothing, demulcent herbs, to recover the energy.

PURGING

Purging, by the use of herbal laxatives, is valuable in treating ailments associated with the presence of excess secretions, buildup of

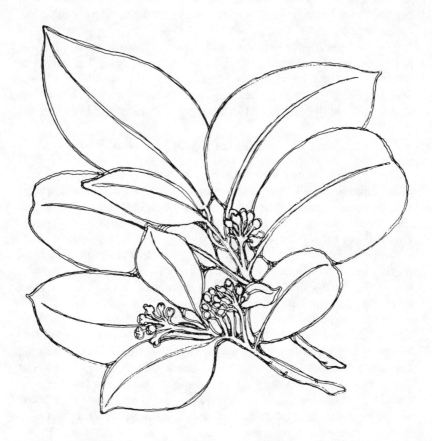

CASCARA SAGRADA (*Rhamnus purshiana*)

One of the safest tonic-laxative herbs known.

toxins or weak elimination. Constipation is considered a serious problem because the retention of wastes in the body can lead to more serious diseases. Purgatives must not be overused, as they deplete the energy of the body, and thus they are only given occasionally to persons who are in relatively good health. Proper elimination is very dependent upon the diet; dietary factors should therefore be emphasized in the regulation of this important function.

Herbs work in a number of ways to promote elimination. Some, like cascara bark and rhubarb root, exert a laxative action by stimulating the secretion of bile into the small intestine and increasing the intestinal peristalsis (the natural rhythmic contractions by which the body moves the intestinal contents along). Others, such as licorice, slippery elm and various oils, are soothing lubricants that have a mild action and may be used to treat minor problems in adults or to treat children. Aloe vera combines both these kinds of actions and may be used for more advanced illnesses accompanied by poor elimination (see "Aloe vera" in the "Herbs to Know" chapter). Bulk laxatives, such as psyllium seed, flax seed and chia seed, swell up with water and work by greatly increasing the bulk in the intestines. These herb seeds are also very nutritive. A combination of these laxative types, for example, with cascara, licorice, psyllium, flax and chia, provides a tonic laxative with nutrients, demulcent properties and stimulation.

Following is a concise table of functions and therapies of the most important herbs.

Herbal Functions and Therapies

HERB (Taken Internally)	Elm.	Mn.	Bld.	St.	Tr.	B.P.	Ton.	Di.	Sw.	Em.	Pur.
Aconite (R)	•	•	•	•	•	•	•	•	•		
Agrimony (W)	•					•	•	•			
Alfalfa (W)	•		•		•	•	•	•			
Aloe (L)	•					•				•	•
Amaranth (W)	•	•				•		•			
Angelica (R)	•	•	•	•		•	•		•		
Anise (S)	•	•		•					•		
Astragalus (R)			•								
Bayberry (B)	•	•		•							
Basil (L)	•	•		•	•	•			•	•	
Bay (L)	•			•							
Blackberry (B)		•	•								
Black cohosh (R)	•	•			•	•		•			
Black pepper (Fr)	•	•		•			•				
Blessed thistle (W)	•	•		•	•	•	•	•	•	•	
Blue cohosh (R)	•	•			•	•		•			
Boneset (W)	•				•	•			•		
Borage (L)	•				•			•			
Buchu (L)	•							•	•		
Burdock (R)	•	•	•			•	•	•	•		
Calamus (R)	•	•	•	•	•						
Calendula (F)	•					•	•		•		
Camomile (F)	•	•	•		•			•	•		
Caraway (S)	•	•		•	•				•		
Cascara (B)	•	•			•		•				•
Catnip (W)	•				•				•		

Elm = Elimination; Mn = Maintenance; Bld = Building; St = Stimulation;
Tr = Tranquilization; BP = Blood Purification; Ton = Tonification;
Di = Diuresis; Sw = Sweating; Em = Emesis; Pur = Purging

HERB (Taken Internally)	FUNCTIONS			THERAPIES							
	Elm.	Mn.	Bld.	St.	Tr.	B.P.	Ton.	Di.	Sw.	Em.	Pur.
Cayenne (*Fr*)	•	•		•	•				•		
Chaparral (*L*)	•					•		•			
Chia (*S*)	•		•			•					•
Chickweed (*W*)	•				•	•		•			
Chrysanthemum (Ch. *F*)		•			•	•					
Cinnamon (*B*)	•	•	•	•			•		•		
Cleavers (*W*)	•					•		•			
Cloves (*F*)	•	•		•	•				•		
Coltsfoot (*L*)	•				•			•			
Comfrey (*L,R*)	•	•	•		•	•	•	•	•		
Coriander (*S*)	•	•		•			•				
Crampbark (*B*)	•	•			•						
Damiana (*L*)	•	•			•	•	•	•			
Dandelion (*L,R*)	•	•	•			•	•	•			•
Dong quai (*R*)			•		•	•	•				
Don sen (*R*)			•	•			•				
Echinacea (*R*)	•	•				•					
Elder (*F*)	•				•	•		•	•		
Elecampane (*W*)	•	•			•		•		•		
Eleutherococcus (*R*)	•		•			•	•				
Ephedra (*W*)	•	•			•				•		
Eucalyptus (*L*)	•				•						
Eyebright (*W*)		•				•	•				
False unicorn (*R*)	•		•	•			•	•			
Fennel (*S*)	•				•	•					
Fenugreek (*S*)	•	•	•		•		•	•			
Flax (*S*)	•	•	•		•	•	•				•
Fu ling (*W*)	•	•	•		•		•	•			
Garlic	•	•	•	•	•	•	•	•	•		

L = leaf; *W* = aboveground portion; *R* = root or rhizome; *S* = seed;
F = flower; *Fr* = fruit; *G* = gum; *B* = bark; Ch = Chinese; J = Japanese.

HERB (Taken Internally)	FUNCTIONS			THERAPIES							
	Elm.	Mn.	Bld.	St.	Tr.	B.P.	Ton.	Di.	Sw.	Em.	Pur.
Gentian (R)		•	•			•	•				
Ginger (R)	•	•		•	•			•	•		
Ginseng (R)			•	•	•		•				
Goldenseal (R)	•	•	•	•	•	•	•	•		•	•
Gota kola (W)	•			•	•	•	•				
Gravelroot (R)	•	•			•			•			
Hawthorn (Fr)	•	•	•		•		•	•			
Honeysuckle (J,F)		•				•					
Hops (L)	•	•			•		•	•			
Horsetail (W)	•				•			•			
Ho shou wu (R)	•	•	•				•	•			
Hyssop (L)	•			•	•			•	•		
Ipecac	•							•		•	
Irish moss (W)			•				•				
Juniper (Fr)	•			•				•			
Kava kava (R)	•	•			•	•	•	•			
Kelp (W)			•				•				
Lady's slipper (R)		•			•						
Lemon balm (L)	•				•			•	•		
Licorice (R)	•	•	•		•	•	•				•
Lily of the valley (R)	•	•	•		•			•	•		
Lobelia (L)	•			•	•					•	
Lycii (Fr)			•				•	•			
Malva (R)		•	•		•	•		•			
Mandrake (R)	•										•
Marjoram (L)	•			•	•			•	•		
Marshmallow (R)		•	•		•	•		•			
Motherwort (W)	•	•			•	•	•	•			
Mugwort (L)	•	•			•		•	•	•		

Elm = Elimination; Mn = Maintenance; Bld = Building; St = Stimulation;
Tr = Tranquilization; BP = Blood Purification; Ton = Tonification;
Di = Diuresis; Sw = Sweating; Em = Emesis; Pur = Purging

HERB (Taken Internally)	FUNCTIONS			THERAPIES							
	Elm.	Mn.	Bld.	St.	Tr.	B.P.	Ton.	Di.	Sw.	Em.	Pur.
Mullein (L)	●	●			●	●		●	●		
Mustard (S)	●			●							
Myrrh (G)	●				●		●	●			
Nettle (L)	●				●	●	●	●	●		
Nutmeg (Fr)	●	●		●			●				
Oregon grape (R)	●	●				●	●	●			●
Pai shu (R)	●						●				
Parsley (L)	●	●		●	●		●	●	●		
Passion flower (W)	●				●		●				
Pennyroyal (W)	●			●	●			●	●		
Peony (R)		●	●			●	●	●			
Peppermint (L)	●			●				●	●		
Plantain (L)	●					●		●			
Poke (R)	●					●				●	●
Prickly ash (B)		●		●				●			
Prince's pine (L)	●					●		●			●
Psyllium (S)	●	●	●				●				●
Raspberry (L)	●			●	●	●		●			
Red clover (F)	●	●			●	●		●			
Rehmania (R)		●	●		●	●	●	●			
Rhubarb (R)	●										●
Rosemary (W)	●			●	●				●		
Rue (L)	●			●	●						
Sage (L)	●			●	●		●	●			
Sarsaparilla (R)	●	●	●			●	●	●	●		
Sassafras (B)	●	●	●	●		●	●	●			
Skullcap (L)	●		●		●	●	●				
Senna (L)	●										●
Slippery elm (B)		●	●			●	●	●			

L = leaf; *W* = aboveground portion; *R* = root or rhizome; *S* = seed; *F* = flower; *Fr* = fruit; *G* = gum; *B* = bark; Ch = Chinese; J = Japanese.

HERB (Taken Internally)	Elm.	Mn.	Bld.	St.	Tr.	B.P.	Ton.	Di.	Sw.	Em.	Pur.
Spearmint (*L*)	•			•	•			•	•		
Squawvine (*L,Fr*)	•	•				•	•	•			
Stoneroot (*R*)	•	•					•	•			
Thyme (*L*)	•			•	•				•		
Tienchi (*R*)		•	•			•	•	•			
Turmeric (*R*)	•	•	•	•		•	•				
Uva ursi (*L*)	•	•				•		•			
Valerian (*R*)		•	•	•	•		•				
Vervain (*W*)	•				•	•		•	•		
White oak (*B*)	•	•				•	•				
Wild cherry (*B*)	•	•				•	•	•			
Wild ginger (*R*)	•			•		•		•	•		
Wild yam (*R*)		•	•		•		•				
Witch hazel (*L*)	•				•		•	•			
Wood betony (*W*)	•	•	•		•		•				
Yarrow (*F*)	•			•	•	•	•	•	•		
Yellow dock (*R*)	•	•					•	•			•
Yerba santa (*L*)	•			•			•		•	•	

Elm = Elimination; Mn = Maintenance; Bld = Building; St = Stimulation;
Tr = Tranquilization; BP = Blood Purification; Ton = Tonification;
Di = Diuresis; Sw = Sweating; Em = Emesis; Pur = Purging
L = leaf; *W* = aboveground portion; *R* = root or rhizome; *S* = seed;
F = flower; *Fr* = fruit; *G* = gum; *B* = bark; *Ch* = Chinese; *J* = Japanese.

4

Methods of Application

In most parts of the world, healers achieve their cures with only a
small variety of plants that are available in the region. Their success
is due not only to their knowledge of these plants, but also to their
ability to administer them in many different ways. One of the most
commonly used preparations is the herbal tea, but there are many
more methods of application, including:

1. bolus;
2. douche;
3. electuary;
4. enema;
5. fomentation;
6. gelatin capsule;
7. liniment;
8. oil;
9. pill;
10. poultice and plaster;
11. salve;
12. smoking;
13. syrup;
14. tincture.

The choice of method will depend on a number of factors; through
familiarity with the nature of the different preparations, one will be
able to choose the method that best fits the ailment, the individual and
the herbs. For quickest results, and especially in treating severe
acute ailments, it will usually be best to take the herbs while fasting

or following a special cleansing diet (see "Therapeutic Diet" suggestions in the "Kitchen Medicines" chapter). The proper use of herbs and diet are certain to strengthen and heal your body if you reduce the intake of toxic or acid-forming foods, get plenty of rest and remove yourself from causes of tension.

MEDICINAL HERB TEAS

Herbs that have a relatively mild flavor and are to be taken internally are frequently taken as an herb tea. When purchasing herbs for making teas, the cut and sifted form is most useful because it is easily strained through any common tea strainer. Fresh herbs are first bruised by rubbing between the hands or using a mortar and pestle to break up the tissue structure and release the active principles. Herbs are prepared in nonmetallic containers such as glass, earthenware or enamel pots. Stainless steel has been found to be acceptable when these others are not available. Use distilled or spring water, rather than tap water, when possible.

There are two basic methods of preparing the tea, infusion and decoction.

Infusion If one is attempting to utilize the volatile oils in herbs such as the mints or eucalyptus, or the delicate plant parts such as flowers and soft leaves, the herbs are steeped in a tightly covered container with water that has just been brought to a rolling boil. This method is called an infusion. The herbs are not boiled at all, but are only steeped, allowing ten to twenty minutes in a tightly covered vessel. A "sun tea" is made by exposing the herbs in water to the sun for a few hours in a tightly covered glass bottle.

Decoction To extract the deeper essences from coarser leaves, stems, barks and roots, the herbs are simmered for about one hour. This method is called a decoction. In many cases, the herbs are simmered uncovered and the volume of water is decreased by about half through evaporation. However, some of these coarser herbs contain important volatile oils, and these must be gently simmered or steeped in a covered pot (valerian, cinnamon and burdock roots, for example).

Combining Decoction and Infusion Occasionally, a formula will combine roots and barks along with soft leaves and flowers. To make a tea, a decoction is first made with the coarser materials, then strained and poured over the delicate plant parts. This is then steeped, tightly covered, for ten to twenty minutes.

Amount to Use Medicinal infusions and decoctions are very strong, and are not like the weak beverage teas familiar to most people. The beverage teas, such as those sold commercially in tea bags, are made using only about one-seventh ounce of herb per pint (two cups) of water. *The usual proportion in making a medicinal tea is one ounce of dried herb per pint of water.* The herb will absorb some of the water, so that after making the tea, perhaps only one and one-half cups of the tea will result from using one pint of water. In most cases, this will be the correct amount for one day, since the therapy usually requires taking one-half cup of the tea, three times daily. For convenience, prepare enough tea for three days of treatment all at once and keep it refrigerated in a tightly closed jar. Herb teas will generally not keep for more than three days in the refrigerator. They should be gently reheated in a covered pot.

If fresh herbs are to be used, the amount is doubled, since much of the weight of the fresh herb is water.

The standard dose of medicinal tea is one-half to one cup taken three times a day. Frequent small doses of two to three tablespoons (taken every half hour) are more effective than a few large doses when treating acute ailments.

In treating chronic ailments where the herbs are to be taken over a period of several weeks, it may be more convenient to use a tincture. Also, if one wishes to restrict the intake of fluids, the tincture will be more useful (see the information on "Diuresis" in the "Herbal Therapies" chapter). Herbs that are mucilagenous, such as slippery elm, comfrey root and marshmallow root, will give the tea a "slimy" quality. If this is disagreeable, the mucilagenous herbs may be put into gelatin capsules or pills and taken along with the tea.

BOLUS

A bolus is a suppository made by adding powdered herbs to cocoa butter until it forms a thick, firm pie-dough consistency. This is placed in the refrigerator to harden and then allowed to warm to room temperature before use. It is rolled into strips about three-quarters of an inch thick and cut into segments one inch long. The bolus is inserted into the rectum to treat hemorrhoids or various cysts, or into the vagina to treat infections, irritations and tumors. The herbs used in the bolus may include astringents such as white oak bark or bayberry bark; demulcent healing herbs such as comfrey root or slippery elm; and antibiotic herbs such as garlic, chaparral or goldenseal. Goldenseal is particularly useful because it is a specific for treating mucous membranes and combines astringent, tissue healing and antibiotic effects.

The bolus is usually applied at night, and the cocoa butter will melt due to the body heat, releasing the herbs. Take precautions to protect clothing and bedding, and rinse away the residue the following morning.

DOUCHE

A douche is generally used in the treatment of vaginal infections or for cleansing. I do not recommend that douches be used often because they disturb the balance of natural bacteria in the vagina. Repeated infections are usually a sign of a poor diet and general lowered resistance of the body.

The douche is made by preparing a strong tea using herbs such as goldenseal, plantain, uva ursi, comfrey, white oak bark or yellow dock. A small amount (one or two tablespoons per quart) of vinegar or yogurt may be added to promote acid balance. The douche is best applied in the bathtub or on the toilet, but never have the bag more than two feet above the hips. The herbal douche is slowly and gently inserted while still warm (body temperature) and retained for a period of ten to twenty minutes, if possible. If the liquid is forced in under too much pressure it may push the infection upward to the uterus. Don't douche if you are pregnant.

ELECTUARY

An electuary is an old-fashioned way of giving unpalatable herbs to children who need them. A small amount of the herb is mixed with honey, maple syrup, peanut butter or other acceptable medium until a soft pasty mass is formed. Small children can even be persuaded to take cayenne in a little peanut butter coated with honey.

ENEMA

Enemas are administered for the treatment of nervousness, pain and conditions associated with excess toxins in the blood. One of the best herbal enemas is catnip tea. Others which are also very useful are those made from a combination of nervines, such as lobelia or skullcap, with astringents, such as yellow dock or bayberry bark. Use equal parts in making a strong tea for use as an enema.

Enemas are given cool (but not cold) if one is trying to remove old waste that has dried and hardened on the intestinal walls. A cool catnip enema is useful to reduce fever. Enemas are given warm for treating nervous conditions.

An enema is taken in first while lying on the left side, then on hands and knees, and finally while lying on the right side. This will help the solution to fill the lower intestines. The herbal fluid is to be retained for as long as possible and the procedure should be repeated during the course of an hour or until two quarts of water can be taken in and retained for a few minutes.

FOMENTATION

A fomentation is an external application of herbs that is used to treat superficial ailments, including swellings, pains, colds and flus. A fomentation can be used to stimulate the circulation of the blood or lymph in the area of the body to which it is applied. Herbs that are too strong to be taken internally may be used externally and the body will absorb a small amount slowly. A fomentation is also known as a compress.

A fomentation is prepared by making an herbal tea, dipping a moisture-absorbent towel or cloth into the tea and applying the towel over the affected area as hot as can be tolerated without burning. The towel is covered by dry flannel cloth and a heating pad or hot water bottle is placed on top of this. A plastic covering is used to protect bedding if applied overnight.

To stimulate circulation of blood and lymph, to relieve colic, to reduce internal inflammation and to restore warmth to cold joints, a ginger fomentation is recommended. Grate two ounces of fresh ginger root and squeeze out the ginger into a pint of hot water until the water turns yellow. Then apply the fomentation, having an alternate towel ready to apply as soon as one cools.

To help restore vitality to a part of the body that has been immobilized or weakened by a disease, the hot fomentation can be alternated with a shorter application of cold. Heat serves to relax the body and open the pores, while cold will stimulate the body and cause contraction. The alternation of hot and cold will revitalize the area.

The value of external herbal application is illustrated by the following experience. A member of my family was suffering from postoperative shock, showing extreme weakness and severe diarrhea. The condition was becoming critical since no nourishment was being assimilated and rapid dehydration was setting in as a result of the diarrhea. The doctors were quite concerned and didn't seem to know what to do. The hospital rules did not permit them to allow me to administer an herb tea that I thought would be of benefit. However, considering it harmless and probably of little effect, they did allow me to apply a hot fomentation of slippery elm tea over the abdomen with a heating pad to keep it warm throughout the night. The next morning, the diarrhea had lessened considerably; dehydration was almost completely stopped; and food was being digested properly. Improvement continued with no further applications of the fomentation being necessary.

GELATIN CAPSULES

Gelatin capsules provide a useful method of taking herbs when the herbs are:
1. to be taken in small amounts (one-half to three grams at a time);
2. bitter-tasting or mucilagenous;
3. to be taken regularly over a long period of time.

There are a variety of capsule sizes, but the most common are the small "0" (single 0) and the larger "00" (double 0) caps. The "00" capsules are generally used unless the capsules are to be taken by children or by someone who finds the larger capsules difficult to swallow. To facilitate washing down and dissolving the capsules, either take them with a meal or drink at least one half to one cup of water or herbal tea.

In many cases, it is necessary to purchase the herb already powdered in order to fill the capsules properly. The herb powdered in a blender or spice grinder may not be fine enough for this purpose. Place the powders in a small bowl and blend them well with a spoon. Separate the two parts of the capsule and press each through the powder to the side of the bowl so that some powder is forced into the capsule. Continue to do this until both ends are almost filled. Then carefully close the capsule. The amount of herb material that fills the capsule will depend on how finely it is powdered, how tightly it is packed and whether it is root, bark, leaf or flower.

Do not use very mild herbs that require large doses to be effective in the capsules. It will not be possible to get an adequate dose this way. Also, do not mix mild acting herbs, except those that are mucilagenous, with more potent herbs in a capsule, since the mild herbs will only dilute the potent herbs and will not be present in sufficient quantity to provide the desired effect.

The typical dose for herbs taken by capsule is two capsules, three times daily, though the actual dose will depend on the herb and the condition being treated. Some herbs, such as goldenseal, mandrake, poke and lobelia, should be taken in much smaller quantities, usually by incorporating them as constituents of a larger formula.

Gelatin capsules may be taken with meals, but if taken between meals *at least one-half cup water or herbal tea should be used to wash them down.*

Whenever a formula calls for using gelatin capsules, one may alternatively make pills, using twice as many pills as capsules to get about the same dose (see the section on "Pills" in this chapter).

LINIMENT

Liniments are herbal extracts that are rubbed into the skin for treating strained muscles and ligaments. They are also used for the relief of arthritis and some types of inflammation. Liniments usually include stimulating herbs, such as cayenne, and antispasmodic herbs, such as lobelia. Oils of aromatic herbs, such as eucalyptus, will penetrate into the muscles, increasing circulation and bringing relaxing warmth to the area.

Place four ounces of dried herbs or eight ounces of fresh bruised herbs into a bottle. Add one pint of vinegar, alcohol or massage oil and allow to extract. Shake the contents of the bottle once or twice a day. The extraction will require three days if the herbs are all powdered, but fourteen days if the herbs are whole or cut.

The vinegar acts as a natural astringent and also as a preservative. It may be used directly or diluted to 50% strength with water. Alcohol is an excellent extracting agent and preservative. One can use a grain alcohol such as vodka or gin, or, if only external use is intended, a rubbing alcohol. The application of the alcohol extract will be somewhat cooling, and the liquid will evaporate quickly leaving the herbal principles in the skin. A massage oil can be made by combining vegetable oils such as olive, sesame and almond. It is useful for extracting herbs with aromatic oils and for applications where one wishes to massage the area being treated. Oils are preserved by adding a small amount of Vitamin E, about 400 IU per cup.

OILS

When the major properties of an herb are associated with its essential oils, an oil extract will prove to be a useful method of preparing a concentrate from fresh herbs. Oils are prepared by macerating and pounding the fresh or dried herbs in a mortar and pestle. Olive oil or sesame oil is then added (one pint oil to two ounces of herb) and the mixture is allowed to stand in a warm place for three days. A quicker method is to gently heat the oil and herbs in a pan for at least one hour. Then the oil is strained and bottled. Yet another method is to extract the herbal properties with alcohol (see the section on "Tinctures" in this chapter), then add the oil and apply gentle heat to evaporate away the alcohol. A small amount of Vitamin E oil (about 400 IU per cup) will help preserve the quality of the preparation.

To obtain an oil made primarily of the essential plant oils, dip thin layers of cotton or cheesecloth in olive or sesame oil, wring out gently and cover each piece with a layer of herbs. Place these pieces of cloth on top of each other in a wide-mouthed jar, covered tightly, for three days and then squeeze out the oil from the cloths.

Oils are frequently made from the spices, mints and other aromatic herbs.

PILLS

Pills are used in the same way as gelatin capsules, but they have the advantage that they can be prepared entirely with herbs and the herbs need not be powdered so finely. Coarse powders can be made from the dried or cut herb using a coffee and spice grinder. To the powdered herbs, add a small amount of slippery elm (or other muci-lagenous herb powder), making up about 10% of the mixture. Slowly add water and mix it in with the herbs until a doughy consistency is reached. Alternatively, one can use a little gum arabic dissolved in boiling water as a good adhesive. Roll the dough into little balls about the size of a pea. The pills may be taken immediately, but to preserve them for later use dry them in the warm air or in an oven at low heat. Strict vegetarians prefer using the pills rather than gelatin capsules, since all available capsules are made from animal gelatin.

The pea-sized pills contain about half the dose of a gelatin capsule. Therefore when following a dosage schedule for gelatin capsules, use twice the number indicated when using pills as a substitute.

POULTICE AND PLASTER

A poultice is a warm, moist mass of powdered or macerated herbs that is applied directly to the skin to relieve inflammation, blood poisoning, venomous bites and eruptions and to promote proper cleansing and healing of the affected area. Many poultices have the power to draw out infection, toxins and foreign bodies embedded in the skin; these usually include comfrey, plantain or marshmallow. To relieve pain and muscle spasm, herbs such as lobelia, lady's slipper, catnip, valerian, kava kava or echinacea are used. Usually a small amount of herbal stimulant, such as ginger or cayenne, is added to promote good circulation. The powdered herbs are moist-ened with hot water, herbal tea, a liniment or a tincture. Herbs that are not available in powder form may be added by using one of these other extraction methods and then adding it to the powder. A witch hazel extract, available at most drugstores, is useful for this purpose.

In the wilds, a poultice can be made by chewing the fresh herbs, such as plantain, before applying them to the affected area.

A plaster is like a poultice, but the herbal materials are either placed between two thin pieces of linen or are combined in a thick base material and then applied to the skin. A classic mustard plaster is described in the "Medicines in the Spice Rack" section of the "Kitchen Medicines" chapter (see under "Mustard seed"). A very effective plaster for drawing out fever is made by squeezing out the water from tofu and then mashing the tofu together with 20% pastry flour and 5% grated fresh ginger root. This is applied directly to the skin for cooling the area. Tofu is a very useful base for many plasters.

SALVE

A salve, or ointment, is a preparation that can be applied to the skin and remain in place due to its thick consistency. A salve can be made by first preparing an herbal oil, heating it and then adding melted beeswax sufficient to obtain the desired consistency (about one and one-half ounces per pint of oil). The quickest method is to extract the herbs in hot oil, allowing about two hours for roots and barks to extract in oil heated to just below the point where it will bubble. Keep the pot covered. Add leaves and flowers next, and continue to cook gently for another hour. Then add the melted wax and stir well. Alternatively mix one part of the powdered herbs into four parts of hot lard or other fat that is hard at room temperature. With either method, add a small amount of gum benzoin or tincture of benzoin to the salve to help preserve it (about one teaspoon of the tincture per quart of salve).

SMOKING

For direct treatment of coughs and bronchial congestion, some herbs are smoked. This will provide immediate, but temporary, relief for the condition. Unlike tobacco, the herbs which are smoked for thera-peutic purposes contain no nicotine or other addicting substances.

A small amount of the herb is smoked in a pipe, or a water pipe. The lungs are filled with smoke and then this is fully exhaled. Inhale the smoke about six to ten times for a single treatment.

The most commonly used herbs that are smoked are coltsfoot, rosemary, mullein, yerba santa and sarsaparilla. To aid in quitting smoking tobacco, lobelia, also known as Indian tobacco, is smoked. It contains lobeline, which is similar to nicotine but does not have the same set of effects. Thus it reduces the sensation of need for

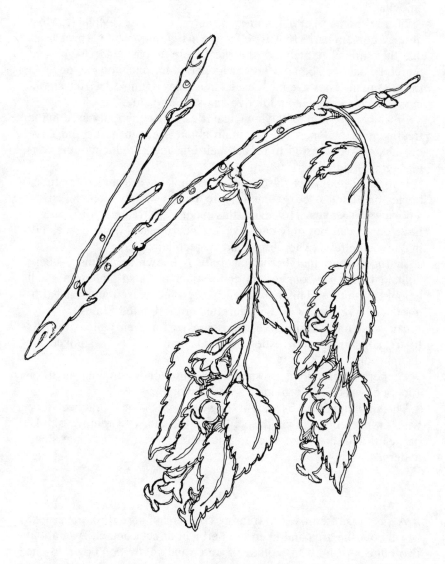

Slippery Elm (*Ulmus fulva*)

Soothing, nutritive and an excellent binder for pills, lozenges and boluses.

nicotine, but does not provide the effects that lead to addictive smoking.

There are a number of commercial herbal cigarettes available. Most of these contain herbs that are effective in treating bronchial problems, but they are also blended specifically for a particular flavor and therefore may not be as useful as an herbal formula you can develop for treatment. They are most useful in making a transition from smoking tobacco to stopping addictive smoking altogether.

In China, "Asthma Allaying Cigarettes" are commonly used in the treatment of asthma. They contain about a dozen herbs and have been extensively tested to reveal their efficacy in reducing lung congestion and aiding expectoration.

Datura stramonium, also known as jimsonweed and giant thorn apple, has been used extensively to treat asthma, often taken by smoking the leaves. However, this plant is extremely toxic and in large doses can not only cause severe neurological disturbances but may even be fatal. Therefore it is not recommended.

In India, a popular herbal cigarette is known as "Bidis." These contain herbs for coughs and congestion, but also include a small amount of datura. This has recently been recognized and has led to a reduced availability of the cigarettes in the United States.

Mugwort and catnip have been smoked for their calming effects to treat insomnia and restlessness. Damiana has been smoked for its aphrodisiac effects.

Peppermint is added to smoking blends for its cooling menthol. Licorice is added to provide a sweet flavor.

The smoking of herbs should only be an occasional practice, done with proper concern for the ability of the lungs to remove smoke particles and tars that are an inevitable result of burning plant materials.

SYRUPS

A syrup is often used in treating coughs and sore throats because it will coat the area and keep the herbs in direct contact. Add about two ounces of herb to a quart of water and gently boil down to one pint. Strain, and while warm, add one or two ounces of honey and/or glycerine. Licorice and wild cherry bark are two herbs commonly used both as flavors and as therapeutic agents in making syrups. Other herbs commonly used in cough syrups are thyme, comfrey root, anise seed, fennel seed, Irish moss and small amounts of lobelia. The syrups are used in doses of one-half to one teaspoon, as needed.

TINCTURES

Tinctures are highly concentrated herbal extracts that can be kept for long periods of time because the alcohol is a good preservative. The final concentration of alcohol in the tincture should not be less than about 30%. Tinctures are particularly useful for herbs that do not taste good or are to be taken over an extended period of time, and they may be used externally as a liniment. Some herbs, such as black cohosh and chaparral, contain substances not readily extracted by water and thus should be taken in pills, capsules or tinctures rather than teas. Alcohol will generally extract all important ingredients from an herb.

To make a tincture, combine four ounces of powdered or cut herb with one pint of alcohol such as vodka, brandy, gin or rum. Shake daily, allowing the herbs to extract for about two weeks. Let the herbs settle and pour off the tincture, straining out the powder through a fine cloth or filter. It is best to put up one's tincture on the new moon and strain it off on the full moon so that the drawing power of the waxing moon will help extract the herbal properties.

The amount of tincture to be taken in a single dose varies from a few drops to two tablespoons. This amount of alcohol is quite small and for most people should not present a problem. If the use of alcohol even at this level must be restricted, the extract may be made with vinegar instead. Tinctures are usually made with the more potent herbs that are generally not taken as herbal teas. If a tincture is to be made with milder herbs, the dose will have to be increased to one or two tablespoons, about the equivalent of one-half cup of the tea.

Do not confuse tinctures with the commercially available "fluid extract." The fluid extract is made by techniques that utilize multiple solvent extraction, resulting in a very concentrated product. These are up to ten times as potent as the tincture and thus are usually taken in quantities of only six to eight drops (the equivalent of a teaspoon of tincture).

The last page of this book provides weights and measures for the preparation of herbal formulas.

5

HERBAL PROPERTIES

The remarkable aspect of herbs is their combination of several different healing properties. Thus each herb will have a combination of specific effects on particular systems of the body, and also some very general effects. By carefully matching the herbal properties with the symptoms being treated, it is possible to confront the entire scope of the disease at once, achieving a cure quickly and with the minimum possible dosage.

Every herb contains hundreds of biochemical constituents that may have an effect on the body. These constituents lend themselves to descriptions according to their physiological effects, or properties. Thus the tannins in many herb plants give rise to the properties "astringent" and "hemostatic," and the aromatic essential oils give rise to such properties as "diaphoretic," "stimulant" and "carminative."

Through the centuries of herbal practice, more than a hundred terms have arisen to describe these properties. Yet there are about three dozen terms that are adequate to describe most herbal effects, after one has eliminated equivalent terms and rarely mentioned properties. These have been included in this chapter to familiarize you with the most frequently considered herbal properties. Many of the same properties have already been referred to in the chapter on "Methods of Application" and will repeatedly be used in the description of the important "Herbs to Know."

Alteratives: Also known as blood purifiers. These are agents that gradually and favorably alter the condition of the body. They are used in treating toxicity of the blood, infections, arthritis, cancer and skin eruptions. Alteratives also help the body to assimilate

40

nutrients and eliminate waste products of metabolism. The choice of alterative depends upon matching the accompanying properties of the herb with the specific nature of the condition being treated. Hence red clover is used to treat cancer because of its effects on protein assimilation; echinacea is used to neutralize acid conditions in the blood associated with a stagnation of lymphatic fluids; sarsaparilla may be used when diuretic properties are needed, as with infections; cascara sagrada is used when a laxative is required, as with toxic conditions resulting from constipation; dandelion root combines hepatic tonic properties and diuretic properties, and is particularly useful for treating chronic problems of blood toxicity; elder flowers have diaphoretic properties, and are thus used to purify the blood during treatment of colds and flus. In addition to the herbs mentioned above, other alteratives include: alfalfa, aloe vera, angelica, burdock root, comfrey, goldenseal, gota kola, marshmallow, nettles, Oregon grape root, plantain, sassafras, uva ursi, chrysanthemum, dong quai, ginseng, ho shou wu, lycii, peony and rehmania.

Analgesics: Herbs that are taken to relieve pain without causing loss of consciousness. Some analgesics are also antispasmodics, relieving pain by reducing cramping in muscles; these include cramp bark and dong quai, which are used to reduce menstrual cramps and associated pain. Others, such as cloves and kava kava, affect the nerves directly, reducing the pain signals to the brain. These may be applied to toothaches for relief. Other analgesics include: lobelia, catnip, camomile, wild yam, skullcap and valerian.

Antacids: Herbs that are able to neutralize excess acids in the stomach and intestines. In most cases, these also have demulcent properties to protect the stomach lining. Dandelion, fennel, slippery elm, Irish moss and kelp function as antacids.

Antiabortives: Herbs that help to inhibit abortive tendencies. These are taken in small quantities during early pregnancy, and include: false unicorn root, lobelia, red raspberry and cramp bark. The herbs will not interfere with the natural process of miscarriage when the fetus is damaged or improperly secured.

Antiasthmatics: Herbs that relieve the symptoms of asthma. Some, like lobelia, are strong antispasmodics that dilate the bronchioles. Others, like yerba santa, help break up the mucus. Some herbs may be smoked for quick relief. These include coltsfoot and mullein, which may also be taken as teas. Other antiasthmatics include: wild yam, comfrey, elecampane and wild cherry bark.

Antibiotics: Substances that inhibit the growth of, or destroy, bacteria, viruses or amoebas. While many herbal antibiotics have direct germ killing effects, they have as a primary action the stimulation of the body's own immune response. Excessive use of antibiotics will eventually destroy the beneficial bacteria of the intestines. In fighting stubborn infections it is a good idea to maintain favorable intestinal flora by eating miso, tamari or fresh yogurt. Important antibiotic herbs include: buchu, chaparral, echinacea, goldenseal, myrrh, juniper berries, thyme and garlic.

Anticatarrhals: Substances that eliminate or counteract the formation of mucus. A treatment for catarrh should also include the use of herbs that aid elimination through sweat (diaphoretics), urine (diuretics) and feces (laxatives). Anticatarrhal herbs include: black pepper, cayenne, ginger, sage, cinnamon, anise, gota kola, mullein, comfrey, wild cherry bark and yerba santa.

Antipyretics: Cooling herbs used to reduce or prevent fevers. Substances with strong cooling properties are called refrigerants. Cooling may refer to neutralizing harmful acids in the blood (excess heat) as well as reducing body temperature. Antipyretics include: alfalfa, boneset, basil, gota kola, skullcap, chickweed and the seaweeds.

Antiseptics: Substances that can be applied to the skin to prevent the growth of bacteria. This includes the astringents. Other antiseptics include: goldenseal, calendula, chaparral, myrrh and the oils of thyme, garlic, pine, juniper berries and sage.

Antispasmodics: Herbs that prevent or relax muscle spasms. They may be applied either internally or externally for relief. One of the most important antispasmodics is lobelia, which has been called the "thinking herb" because it has been used successfully whenever there was any uncertainty as to the method of treatment. Antispasmodics are included in most herb formulas to relax the body and allow it to use its full energy for healing. Other antispasmodics include: dong quai, black cohosh, blue cohosh, skullcap, valerian, kava kava, raspberry leaves and rue.

Aphrodisiacs: Substances used to improve sexual potency and power. Aphrodisiacs include: damiana, false unicorn, ginseng, angelica, astragalus, kava kava and burdock.

Astringents: Substances that have a constricting or binding effect. They are commonly used to check hemorrhages and secretions, and

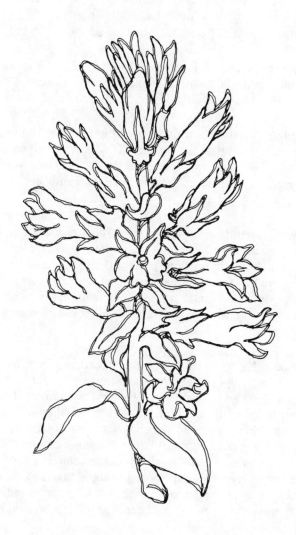

LOBELIA (*Lobelia inflata*)

"The Thinking Herb."
Certain to be valuable whenever an antispasmodic is needed.

to treat swollen tonsils and hemorrhoids. The main herbal astringents contain tannins, which are found in most plants, especially in tree barks. Important astringents include: bayberry bark, white oak bark, yellow dock, uva ursi, calendula, myrrh, horsetail, juniper berries, prince's pine, stoneroot, squawvine and witch hazel.

Carminatives: Herbs and spices taken to relieve gas and griping (severe pains in the bowels). Examples of carminatives include: anise, caraway, fennel, cumin, dill, ginger, peppermint and calamus.

Cholagogues: Substances used to promote the flow and discharge of bile into the small intestine. These will also be laxatives, as the bile will stimulate elimination. Aloe vera, barberry, Oregon grape root, culver's root, mandrake, goldenseal, wild yam and licorice are cholagogues.

Demulcents: Soothing substances, usually mucilage, taken internally to protect damaged or inflamed tissues. Usually a demulcent herb will be used along with diuretics to protect the kidney and urinary tract, especially when kidney stones and gravel are present. Important demulcents include: marshmallow, comfrey, Irish moss, slippery elm, chickweed, licorice, psyllium, flax, chia seeds, aloe vera, burdock and fenugreek.

Diaphoretics: Herbs used to induce sweating. To administer diaphoretics effectively, the stomach and bowels should be emptied by fasting and using an herbal enema. However, laxatives should not be taken before using these herbs. Sweating teas should be taken hot; when given cold they act as diuretics. One must distinguish between relaxing diaphoretics and stimulating diaphoretics (see the "Herbal Therapies" chapter). Relaxing diaphoretics include lemon balm and catnip. Stimulating diaphoretics are generally taken along with other stimulants, such as ginger or cayenne, and include: elder flowers, yarrow flowers, boneset, hyssop, peppermint and blessed thistle.

Diuretics: Herbs that increase the flow of urine. Diuretics are used to treat water retention, obesity, lymphatic swellings, nerve inflammations such as lumbago and sciatica, infections of the urinary tract, skin eruptions and kidney stones. Whenever a diuretic is given, a lesser amount of a demulcent herb is also given to buffer the effect of the diuretic on the kidneys (especially when the diuretic contains irritating properties) and to protect the tissues from the movement of kidney stones. Diuretics include: agrimony, horsetail, parsley, uva ursi, cleavers, buchu, juniper, marshmallow, plantain, nettles, burdock, dandelion, hawthorn and pai shu.

Emetics: Substances that induce vomiting and cause the stomach to empty (see the "Herbal Therapies" chapter). In small quantities these will not cause emesis, but will have other important effects on the body. Lobelia, black mustard seed, ipecac, bayberry, elecampane and blessed thistle are emetics.

Emmenagogues: Herbs that promote menstruation, usually causing it to occur earlier, and sometimes with increased flow. These have been used in the past to induce abortions, but extreme caution is advised. All of these, when taken in sufficient quantity to cause abortion, have other strong effects on the body. None of these should be taken when a woman wants to be pregnant. They are now commonly used to help regulate the menstrual cycle. Herbs with strong emmenagogue properties include: pennyroyal, juniper berries, myrrh, black cohosh, rue, angelica and wild ginger.

Emollients: Substances that are softening, soothing and protective to the skin. These include: oils of almond, apricot kernel, wheat germ, sesame, olive, linseed and flaxseed, and herbs such as marshmallow, comfrey root, slippery elm and chickweed.

Expectorants: Herbs that will assist in expelling mucus from the lungs and throat. Expectorants include: wild cherry bark, coltsfoot, yerba santa, lobelia, mullein, elecampane, horehound and anise. Also, to loosen mucus, inhale steam from boiled water with eucalyptus, bay leaves and sage.

Galactogogues: Substances that increase the secretion of milk. Anise seed, blessed thistle, cumin, fennel and vervain are galactogogues.

Hemostatics: Substances that arrest hemorrhaging. These include astringents and herbs that affect the coagulation of blood. Bayberry, blackberry, cayenne, cranesbill, mullein, goldenseal, horsetail, uva ursi, white oak bark, yellow dock, witch hazel and tienchi are hemostatics.

Laxatives: Substances that promote bowel movements. (See the section on "Purging" in the "Herbal Therapies" chapter for details.) A strong laxative that causes increased intestinal peristalsis is called a purgative in many texts.

Lithotriptics: Herbs that help to dissolve and eliminate urinary and biliary stones and gravel. For the kidney and bladder stones, use gravel root, cleavers, parsley, dandelion, nettle, uva ursi and horsetail. For the gallbladder, use wild cherry bark, Oregon grape root and cascara sagrada.

Nervines: Herbs that calm nervous tension and nourish the nervous system. See *Tonics*.

Oxytocics: Substances that stimulate uterine contractions to assist and induce labor, thus hastening childbirth. Oxytocics include: angelica, black cohosh, blue cohosh, juniper berries, raspberry, rue, squawvine, uva ursi and wild ginger.

Parasiticides: Substances that destroy parasites in the digestive tract or on the skin. Garlic, rue, thyme oil, cinnamon oil and chaparral are parasiticides.

Purgatives: (See *Laxatives*)

Rubefacients: Substances that increase the flow of blood at the surface of the skin and produce redness where they are applied. Their function is to draw inflammation and congestions from deeper areas. They are useful for the treatment of arthritis, rheumatism and other joint problems and for sprains. Rubefacients include: mustard seed oil, cayenne, black pepper, pine oil, thyme oil, eucalyptus, cinnamon and cubeb oil.

Sedatives: Herbs that strongly quiet the nervous system. These will include antispasmodics and nervines. Useful sedatives include: valerian, hops, camomile, kava kava, passion flower, wood betony, catnip and skullcap.

Sialagogues: Substances that stimulate the flow of saliva and thus aid in the digestion of starches. Echinacea, black pepper, cayenne, ginger, licorice and yerba santa are sialagogues.

Stimulants: Herbs that increase the energy of the body, drive the circulation, break up obstructions and warm the body (see the "Herbal Therapies" chapter). Stimulants include: anise, cayenne, black pepper, cinnamon, echinacea, ginseng, sarsaparilla, dandelion, elecampane, angelica, ginger, yarrow, rosemary, garlic, onion, juniper berries, sage, pennyroyal, bayberry bark and astragalus.

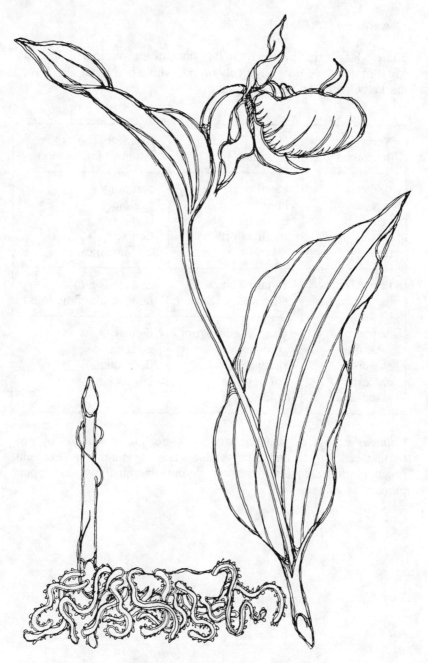

LADY'S SLIPPER (*Cypredium pubescens*)

One of the purest and surest-acting nervines.

Stomachics (see *Tonics*)

Tonics: Herbs that promote the functions of the systems of the body. Most tonics have general effects on the whole body, but also have a marked effect on a specific system.

Nerve Tonics (nervines)	Heart Tonics (cardiac tonics)	Stomach Tonics (stomachics, bitters)
skullcap lobelia valerian lady's slipper fu ling	hawthorn lily of the valley ginseng motherwort rehmania	agrimony gentian barberry don sen elecampane
Liver Tonics (hepatics)	Biliary Tonics (stimulates bile)	Sexual Tonics (aids sexual functions)
dandelion sassafras stoneroot cascara mandrake	Oregon grape root goldenseal rhubarb parsley wild yam	damiana ginseng dong quai burdock licorice

Vulneraries: Herbs that encourage the healing of wounds by promoting cell growth and repair. Aloe vera, cayenne, comfrey, fenugreek, garlic, calendula, rosemary, thyme, marshmallow and slippery elm act as vulneraries.

6

DIAGNOSIS AND TREATMENT

It is much more important to know what sort of patient has a disease than what sort of disease a patient has.

— SIR WILLIAM OSLER

Until the advent of modern medicine, diagnosis and treatment were based on four things:
1. a general theory of health and disease;
2. an intuitive appraisal of the patient's condition and the nature of the curative agents;
3. directing the patient towards making those changes necessary to promote self-healing;
4. experience.

More recently the theory of health has been all but lost, and only pathology is studied; intuition is often replaced by distant analysis; the role of "healing" is placed on the drug or on physical intervention (surgery, radiation, etc.); and experience has been replaced by a continuous onslaught of new synthetic drugs and physical techniques that nature never counted on in the evolution of the human body.

There are a number of traditional medicine systems that provide a pathway to a better interaction between patient and healer and to the active participation of the patient in healing his/her disease. These many traditions differ primarily in the particulars of the theory of health and disease and in the curative agents available to them. All rely on the idea of balance in health, and disease as a reflection of imbalance. All rely on an intuitive approach to diagnosis and treatment.

The diagnosis is an integral part of the treatment. As was mentioned earlier, an ailment provides a focal point for discovering all the negative energies we have cultivated. The diagnosis, which is an unveiling of these negative energies, provides direct and immediate knowledge of how to stop feeding the disease process. This knowledge is the first step in healing oneself.

The Chinese system of diagnosis and treatment, with a 5,000 year history of proven efficacy, is still in use today not only in China, but throughout the Orient. It is particularly valuable for us to use in understanding and practicing herbal medicine. Its universal appeal has led to many of its practices being widely accepted, and much effort has already gone into making the theories available to students in the West.

The most important aspect of the Chinese system to understand in beginning to practice diagnosis and treatment is the science of Yin and Yang.

The Yin/Yang theory is a teaching method and does not define anything absolute. It shows the way to develop a valuable intuition in diagnosis and treatment. Thus it is important to avoid getting attached to the symbols Yin and Yang, for they are only tools.

Yin and Yang represent the two essential opposites that make up all opposites. Thus dark/light, cold/hot, wet/dry, in/out, etc., are examples of opposites that we can use to classify and describe our observations. We can see several aspects of these opposites that provide a basis for Yin/Yang theory:

1. the terms are relative and there is a continuous variation between the extremes suggested by the terms;
2. as one condition increases, its opposite decreases (with more heat, there is less cold);
3. everything undergoes change, and the description of anything by these opposites must change in time;
4. the opposites may be grouped together to form two sets based on our experience. For example, think of a dark, cold, wet basement versus a sunny, hot, dry desert.

In terms of health and disease, a number of pairs of opposites can be utilized to gain an insight into diagnosis and treatment based on our everyday experience of the world. A few that are particularly useful are:

Yin	*Yang*
cold	hot
wet	dry
deficiency	excess
deep	superficial

The terms on the left represent the typical Yin-type conditions and those on the right represent the typical Yang-type conditions. In the process of diagnosis, one looks for Yin-like or Yang-like conditions in both the basic constitution of the person and in the nature of the ailment. The chart of Yin conditions and Yang conditions shows examples of characteristics you might find present.

Yin Conditions

COLD:	poor circulation; cold hands and feet; subnormal fevers; muscle cramps and spasms; desire for warmth
DEFICIENCY:	anemia; vitamin, mineral or protein deficiencies; underweight; paleness; clear urine; low vitality; timidity; shallow, weak breath; fatigue and tiredness
DEEP:	involves internal organs; sensitive emotional states; tolerates or prefers deep massage
WET:	history of eating raw fruits and vegetables; frequent urination; watery stools containing undigested foods; thin, clear mucus
OTHER DIAGNOSTIC FEATURES	pulse feels slow, deficient, weak, sunken or deep; tongue appears pale, lightly coated

Yang Conditions

HOT:	inflammatory; high fevers; burning sensation; irritability; desire for cool things; hot hands and feet
EXCESS:	rapid breathing; loud, coarse speech; forceful; high blood pressure; insomnia; overweight; red face; cloudy urine
SUPERFICIAL:	acute ailments; ailments due to exposure to cold, damp wind; aversion to deep massage or pressure on the abdomen
DRY:	constipation, dry mouth; mucus is thick (white, yellow or tinged with blood); history of eating meat
OTHER DIAGNOSTIC FEATURES:	pulse feels rapid, forceful, full; tongue is heavily furred, coated white, yellow, red or purple

One rarely sees purely Yin or purely Yang conditions but rather a combination of both. In order to determine the nature of the ailment and the best treatment it is necessary to look at the primary diagnostic concerns. *For acute ailments, consider the most serious symptoms; for chronic ailments, consider the basic constitution and behavior of the individual.*

In general, an individual with a Yang-type constitution and diet will have Yang-type ailments and a Yin-type constitution will be associated with Yin-type ailments. However, this is not always the case, and a severe excess of Yin or Yang character can cause what are called "false-Yin" or, more commonly occurring, "false-Yang" diseases. As an example, one who is thin, weak, complains of coldness and eats a primarily vegetarian diet would be considered to have a Yin constitution. However, due to the extreme imbalance, this person may suffer from a disease with a thick yellowish discharge from the lungs and a high fever, both characteristic of a Yang-type ailment. This is called a false-Yang disease and is treated by providing herbs specific for congestion and fever (treating the acute symptoms) along with a diet to bring the Yin condition back to balance (treating the chronic deficiency).

The method of treating an imbalance of Yin and Yang constitution is to provide a diet and herbal therapy that provides more of the Yin or Yang nature that is lacking. Hence those with a Yin constitution are given a diet and herbs with somewhat more Yang character than they usually use, and those with a Yang constitution are given a diet and herbs with somewhat more Yin character. It is important to avoid using foods and herbs that are extremely Yin or extremely Yang, as it is almost impossible to obtain a good balance that way. Rather, one should use substances that are themselves in balance.

The chart on page 68 indicates the relative Yin and Yang qualities of common foods and herbs.

Qualities of foods and herbs that represent the Yin character include cool, moist or liquid, light, sweet and sour. Generally the Yin substances help stimulate the process of elimination rather than building. The Yin herbs are the flowers, leaves and soft stems.

Qualities of foods and herbs that represent the Yang character include dryness, concentrated protein, saltiness, mild sweetness, bitter flavors and growing under the ground. Meat and fish are considered Yang substances and of the plants, the roots, bark or hard branches are considered more Yang. These generally aid in the process of building the body.

Foods

MORE YIN			BALANCED					MORE YANG
Watery Fruits	Small Fruits	Leaves	Roots	Seeds	Dairy	Fish	Poultry	Red Meat
orange	cherry	spinach	carrot	rice	cheese	cod	chicken	pork

Herb Tonics

MORE YIN			BALANCED			MORE YANG
Small Fruits	Flowers	Leaves	Neutral Roots and Barks	Bitter Roots and Barks	Long Roots	Processed Roots
hawthorn	camomile	comfrey	echinacea	rhubarb	dandelion	rehmania
juniper	honeysuckle	alfalfa	eleuthero	gentian	burdock	red ginseng
lycii	elder	skullcap	slippery elm	cascara	ginseng	aconite (Ch)

A very general layout of foods and herb tonics according to basic Yin/Yang qualities. There are exceptions.

Foods and herbs that are more Yin in quality can be balanced by preparing them in such a way as to introduce or accentuate Yang qualities and vice versa. Yang qualities are provided by adding heat (increasing the cooking time), by drying, by adding a little salt or by cooking with pressure. Yin qualities may be provided by adding water, by reducing the cooking time, by adding honey or other sweeteners, by adding vinegar or by cooling. Thus a very Yin food, such as a tomato, can be made more balanced by cooking it for a very long time and reducing the moisture through evaporation. A Yang food, such as chicken, can be made more balanced by adding water and making chicken soup.

The foods and herbs that are most balanced include grains, beans, seeds and roots. Therefore, these should make up the bulk of the diet and treatment for most individuals. Substances having somewhat more Yin or more Yang quality may be used to aid in the shift towards the balance point and are used in addition to those foods and herbs that are balanced in themselves. Of course, the Yin and Yang qualities of both foods and herbs represent only one aspect of their effects on the body, and the various nutrients and properties are also of great importance.

7

A BALANCED DIET

A good and proper diet in disease is worth a hundred
medicines and no amount of medication can do good to
a patient who does not observe a strict regimen of diet.
— CHARAKA SAMHITA (ca. 300 A.D.)

Diet is the essential key to all successful healing. Without a proper balanced diet, the effectiveness of herbal treatment is very limited. With the appropriate eliminative or balanced diet, herbal treatment will prove itself to be effective where no other medicine will work and will often be faster than the quick but temporary relief offered by Western drugs.

The nutritional philosophy I have found to be the best and easiest centers around the use of whole grains, properly cooked foods and small amounts of fresh vegetables and fruits when they are in season. This basic dietary approach is the foundation of traditional ethnic diets of people around the world and is summarized by the principles of Yin/Yang described in the previous chapter.

To construct a simple balanced diet, the intake of foods can be divided into three categories:

PRIMARY FOODS: whole grains (and a lesser amount of beans to balance protein) make up 40–60% of the diet

SECONDARY FOODS: fresh vegetables, in season, mostly cooked, make up 30–40% of the diet

TERTIARY FOODS: meat, dairy and fruits make up not more than 10–20% of the diet

The primary foods are in themselves balanced in Yin/Yang qualities. Brown rice (the most balanced), millet, wheat, barley, oats, corn, rye and buckwheat and many more whole grains are true energy foods. Beans, especially black and aduki beans, and soybean products such as tofu and miso, are useful in providing a balance of protein when used in combination with the grains. Eating bread is generally not a good method of obtaining the value of grains because it is usually gulped and thus not adequately predigested by saliva. If bread is used, it should be very well chewed.

These primary foods are an essential part of a healing treatment. When American doctors and scientists went to the jungles of Mexico to study the herbal medicines used by the highly reputed curanderos (healers), they verified that many diseases they had considered difficult or impossible to cure were being successfully treated. Upon applying the same treatments here, they were unable to achieve good results and eventually abandoned the treatments. However, when one doctor returned to watch more carefully and determine the basis of the curanderos' effectiveness, he discovered that the patients, without any prompting on the part of the healer, would go on a restricted diet, eating only cornmeal. In fact, the young Indian children were fed only corn and whole grains up to the age of eight years to prevent spoiling their tastes and so that in the event of sickness it would be easy for them to go on this restricted diet. This, he reasoned, was certainly the factor that was missed when the herbal medicines were tried elsewhere.

The secondary foods are fresh, local, seasonal vegetables, which provide important vitamin and mineral nutrients. These foods, however, are somewhat Yin (those eaten raw or cold being more Yin, and those cooked being more balanced) and stimulate the process of elimination. Elimination is an important process, since the proper removal of waste and toxins, either ingested or produced through normal metabolism, is essential for health. Excessive use of these foods will lead to overelimination, leaving the body weak and cold, often with excess water. Therefore these foods should make up only 30–40% of the diet. In therapy, where elimination of toxins is called for and where the individual has been eating too much meat and processed foods, vegetables such as fresh salads are useful in the detoxification needed to begin healing. The most valuable vegetables are the seaweeds, such as hiziki, dulse, kelp, wakame, arame and Irish moss. These are very high in essential minerals and vitamins.

The third level of foods are those we can easily get by with eating very little, or none, of. They include the very Yin foods (fruits) and the very Yang foods (meat and eggs).

Fruits are eliminative and cooling to the body. In small amounts they may be used for these purposes, and thus fruit is usually taken in the middle of the day, when the internal and external temperatures are highest. Fruits taken in the cold of morning or night overcool the body and lead to imbalance of the organ systems. Excessive use of fruits will lead to weakness and deficiencies through their strong eliminative function. A small amount of baked fruits or cooked dried fruits may be taken to stimulate elimination more mildly.

Meat, eggs and dairy are high protein foods, which are building but lack fiber, an important element in digestion and elimination. They are very Yang in quality and provide strong stimulation to the organ systems. Excessive use of these foods leads to overweight, buildup of toxins (especially uric acid from excess protein intake) and poor elimination. Small amounts, especially when taken with vegetables or as a soup, are useful in building after a debilitating illness or after excessive elimination resulting from a diet rich in raw fruits and vegetables.

A balanced diet will also be a low cost diet. Grains, beans and local vegetables in season are the cheapest food items. Exotic fruits and vegetables imported from distant climates will throw us off balance at a high price. There are also specific items to avoid: white sugar, denatured flour and artificial stimulants. These drain the energy of the body and make the assimilation of nutrients from whole foods more difficult. Thus the best diet is one that bypasses the recent technological changes in food supply and relies on nature for its health-giving qualities.

8

KITCHEN MEDICINES

Herbs as Sources of Vitamins and Minerals

Most of us suffer from deficiencies in some vitamins and minerals. These deficiencies are not resolved by taking expensive food supplements, most of which are rapidly eliminated through the urine and wasted. This is because the deficiency is due to imbalance and poor assimilation or rapid elimination of these important nutrients. (Persons with diets consisting primarily of fruits and vegetables will excessively eliminate minerals and vitamins from the system, despite the high intake accompanying these foods. Persons with a diet rich in meats will fail to absorb the necessary nutrients from the food because the digestive and absorptive functions become separated with this kind of diet.) Adding large doses of purified vitamins and minerals will generally fail to overcome these problems.

The key to total nutrition is a balanced diet. Herbs are useful as a part of the balanced diet and also as an aid in remedying a long-term nutritional deficiency. This is done in two ways:

1. the tonic herbs improve the assimilation of vital nutrients by the organs (sometimes referred to as a "Yang tonic");
2. the nutritive herbs provide substantial amounts of balanced minerals and vitamins in a form that is easy to assimilate (sometimes referred to as "Yin tonics").

The most important herbs for providing nutrients are the seaweeds (kelp, Irish moss, etc.), the docks (yellow dock) and dandelion. The most important herbs for providing vitamins are parsley leaves, dandelion leaves and alfalfa.

60

HERBAL SEASONING FOR VITAMINS AND MINERALS

Combine one part each of the culinary herbs (garlic, parsley, watercress, sweet basil, oregano, marjoram and thyme), using whatever is readily available. Add one part each of kelp powder, dulse powder, nettles, comfrey, rose hips and capsicum. Then add one-quarter part each dandelion root powder and burdock root powder. Make a small amount of the blend and then adjust to taste.

MINERAL FORMULA

A formula to supply easily assimilated minerals such as iron, calcium, silicon, magnesium, potassium, sulfur, iodine, zinc, magnesium and trace minerals. Good for all deficient and anemic conditions. Take:

> Parsley root and leaf
> Yellow dock
> Nettles
> Irish moss
> Horsetail
> Comfrey root
> Watercress
> Kelp

Simmer slowly *equal* parts of these herbs, four ounces to a quart of water. Continue to simmer until volume of liquid is reduced by half. Strain, keep the liquid and cover the herbs with water once more; simmer again for ten minutes. Strain again and combine the two liquids. Cook this down until the volume is reduced by half. Add an equal amount of blackstrap molasses. Dosage: take one tablespoon, three to four times daily.

Therapeutic Diet

At the first sign of acute disease one should abstain from all solid foods. In general, the diet should be wholesome, light, warm, easily digested and mostly liquid during the acute crisis. One should avoid heavy, hard-to-digest foods such as meat, cheese and bread. It is also important to avoid excess use of fruits and raw vegetables. Light soups and the appropriate herb teas should be taken. For those who need to eliminate toxins from a meat diet, some warm fruit juice can be taken.

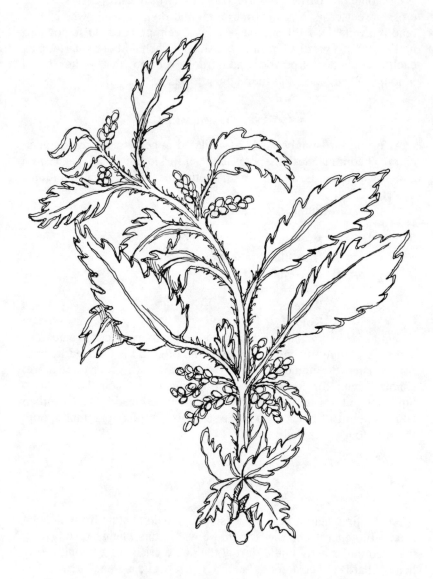

NETTLES (*Urtica urens*)

Rich in minerals and an aid to the assimilation of minerals.

KICHAREE

As one's condition improves, more solid foods can be added to the diet in the form of steamed vegetables and soupy grains. Miso soup and Kicharee are also useful foods. Kicharee is made by mixing one-half cup mung beans or lentils with one-half cup brown rice and sautéing in sesame oil or clarified butter (ghee) for five minutes with a pinch of cumin seed, one-third teaspoon turmeric and one teaspoon ground coriander. Then add four cups of water and simmer for twenty to twenty-five minutes. If desired this can be topped with a small amount of yogurt. Kicharee is well balanced and high in easily assimilated protein. It also has blood purifying properties.

GHEE

Ghee is clarified butter, a delicious and fragrant oil that is semi-liquid at room temperature. It is very useful in cooking and makes an excellent base for herbal salves and oils. To make ghee, melt two pounds of butter in a saucepan until it reaches a slow, rolling boil. Remove from the heat and carefully skim off the foam with a spoon. Return the pot to the heat and repeat this procedure twice more, removing as much of the foam as possible and discarding it. Allow the pan to cool two minutes and then remove a thin film that forms. Let the butter cool down somewhat, and then, while still liquid, pour through a fine-meshed tea strainer, but stop pouring when the heavier solids at the bottom of the pan move to the strainer. Collect the ghee in a glass bottle, cool completely and cover. The whole process takes about twenty minutes. Two pounds of butter will yield about one pound of ghee. It can be stored without refrigeration for six months.

FOUR DAY CLEANSING FAST

Fasting is done for a number of reasons; among them are:
1. as a way of becoming more sensitive to the body;
2. for a curative effect, especially with chronic ailments;
3. to lose excess weight or excess water;
4. to clean out accumulated wastes;
5. to free the blockages of energy flow in the body;
6. for longevity;
7. as a way of developing calmness, control and will power.
A four day cleansing fast is adequate to satisfy these concerns for most people. The method of fasting will depend on the nature of the usual diet and the constitution of the individual. For persons whose

diet is high in meat and for those with a predominantly Yang constitution, the cleansing through "expansion" is most suitable. This
relies on stimulating the process of elimination, especially through
the bowels. For persons whose diet is predominantly vegetarian and
for those with a Yin constitution, the cleansing through "contraction"
is used. This method relies primarily on removing water from the
system.

Expansion The first three days of the fast are begun each morning
with an herbal enema using a tea of raspberry, comfrey or catnip
leaf. Then one or two eight ounce glasses of prune juice can be taken
to stimulate elimination and to help draw the toxins down into the
bowels. Every two hours throughout the day, drink a glass of fresh
apple juice. To stimulate the secretion of bile and elimination of toxins,
one should take a tablespoon of olive oil with one-half teaspoon of
cayenne (one "00" capsule) two to four times per day. Persons who
are overweight but who are not weakened may also use the weight
loss formula (see the "Treatments for Specific Ailments" chapter).

On the fourth day, one begins to break the fast, and after the enema
and prune juice, a lunch of some lightly cooked (steamed or baked)
fruits or vegetables can be taken. Soupy grains may then be added,
and a balanced normal diet can be resumed on the fifth day.

Contraction Begin each day of the fast with an herbal enema using a
tea of raspberry, comfrey or catnip leaf. Eat a small bowl of brown
rice three times a day with no additional liquids. For a more effective
fast, eat only one bowl of rice a day, taking a tablespoon whenever
there is strong hunger, chewing it very well. No other foods or drinks
are to be taken during the four day fast. However, this method of
fasting may cause a mild constipation and if this occurs a small bowl
of stewed prunes may be taken once each day.

To break the fast, on the fifth day, take only lightly cooked fruits
and vegetables, and soupy grains. Resume a normal balanced diet,
high in grains, on the sixth day.

This diet is very good for eliminating excess moisture, reducing
coldness of the body and restoring the ability to assimilate nutrients.
It will also help remove the sensation of excessive thirst for those who
normally experience that condition.

Alternating Expansion and Contraction Either method of fasting may
precipitate a minor healing crisis. If one does not obtain significant
changes in condition or experience a healing crisis, it may be useful to

use the opposite cleansing method. Sometimes it is necessary to alternate between expansion and contraction to encourage the body to dump its toxic wastes.

HEALING CRISIS

The healing crisis is recognized in all systems of natural healing. The Chinese refer to this as the "law of cure." It is not uncommon with effective therapy that one seems to get worse before getting better. When the body is engaged in the elimination of toxins accumulated over the years, one may experience aches, pains and symptoms of diseases, from the most recent to those of childhood. This is because the toxins are being liberated from their storage places and are now actively affecting the body with full force. This is the healing crisis.

If you experience discomfort or marked weakness during the four day fast or as a result of taking the herbs and recommended diet, you should strengthen your determination to go through with it. Strength and improved well-being will return when the process of elimination has been sufficiently accomplished. The cleansing fast can be repeated after one month to help complete the process.

Medicines in the Spice Rack

A convenient place to discover the medicinal value of herbs is the kitchen spice shelf. The common culinary herbs and spices so often added to foods for flavor also have considerable medicinal use and it is likely that they were originally added to foods for these reasons as well.

Most herbal spices are carminatives (preventing and relieving gas), stimulants and aids to digestion. Many of them are also used to relieve nervousness, spasms and coldness. They are often regarded as "crisis medicine," being useful for the first acute stages of disease. Thus the kitchen spice shelf can be thought of as a safe and natural alternative to the synthetic drugs found in the medicine cabinet. Spices can be used to treat problems ranging from bleeding, diarrhea and headache to heart attacks and acute infections.

Anise *(Pimpinella anisum)*
Anise is very useful for breaking up mucus and is thus used for hard dry coughs where expectoration is difficult. A tea is made by

adding a cup of boiled water to three teaspoonsful of crushed seeds, steeping for twenty minutes, and sweetening with a little honey. The tea may be used to stimulate the production of mother's milk. The seeds may also be smoked or added to a cough syrup formula (see the "Methods of Application" chapter).

It is also used as a stimulant and carminative to treat flatulence and colic, taken as a tea. Added to laxative formulas, it will reduce griping (cramping of the bowels).

Basil *(Ocimum basilicum)*

Sweet basil is good to use as a tea for indigestion, fevers, colds, flu, kidney and bladder troubles, headaches, cramps, nausea, vomiting, constipation and nervous conditions. Its medicinal properties include carminative, antipyretic, stimulant, alterative, diuretic and nervine. A tea made of one ounce basil leaves to a pint of water simmered for twenty minutes with three powdered black peppercorns per cup will be effective for most fevers.

Bay *(Laurus nobilis)*

The bay tree was dedicated by the ancient Greeks to Apollo and Aesculapius, the god of medicine. Bay was considered capable of increasing and maintaining health and happiness. One or two bay leaves added to soup and beans improves the flavor and also helps prevent gas and indigestion. They are too strong to be used in large amounts internally, but externally the leaves can be applied as a poultice on the chest with a cloth covering to relieve bronchitis and coughs. Oil of bay, which is made by heating the leaves in a little olive oil, can be applied with great benefit to rheumatic and arthritic aches and pains as well as to swellings and sprains.

Black Pepper *(Piper nigrum)*

Black pepper is an excellent remedy one can take at the first sign of most diseases. Yogis consider black pepper to be one of nature's most perfect foods and useful not only to cure disease but also as a preventive, taking a dose of seven peppercorns ground (one-eighth teaspoon powder) and mixed with honey each morning. The mixture of pepper and honey is useful to overcome cold mucous diseases and sore throats. When treating acute diseases it may be used three to four times a day.

Caraway *(Carum carvi)*

Caraway is an excellent aid to digestion. It is taken for indigestion, gas, colic and nervous conditions. An ounce of the crushed seeds are used in making a pint of the infusion, using boiled water and steeping twenty minutes, or letting the seeds stand in cold water overnight. The tea is then taken in frequent doses of two tablespoons until relief is obtained. Caraway is a mild stimulant and may be added to herb formulas for digestion and laxative formulas to prevent griping.

Cardamom *(Elettaria cardamomum)*

Cardamom is a carminative and stimulant commonly mixed with other spices to treat indigestion and gas. It warms the body and is good for diarrhea, colic and headaches. It is an important ingredient in Chai tea, an Indian spice tea valued for its warm, stimulating effects. To make this tea, grate one ounce of fresh ginger, add seven peppercorns, a cinnamon stick, five cloves and fifteen cardamom seeds and heat in one pint of water, simmering for ten minutes. Then add one-half cup of milk and simmer for another ten minutes. Add a sprinkle of nutmeg and a few drops of vanilla extract. Drink one cup of the tea, sweetened with honey, twice per day or as needed for warmth.

Cayenne *(capsicum anuum)*

The genus Capsicum includes red and green chilies, cayenne, paprika and bell peppers. Cayenne originated in Central and South America where it was extensively used by the natives for many diseases, including diarrhea and cramps.

Cayenne is a stimulant, astringent, carminative and antispasmodic, and is considered a superior crisis herb, useful as a first aid remedy for most conditions. Taken as a daily tonic, one-quarter teaspoon three times daily, it is of benefit for the heart and circulation, preventing heart attack, strokes, colds, flu, diminished vitality, headaches, indigestion, depression and arthritis.

Since cayenne is so hot, the idea that it will not be harmful is sometimes difficult for a beginning user to believe. However, I have used it hundreds of times as often as one teaspoon every fifteen minutes during a crisis and there has never been any problem. On the contrary, it helped to effect a speedy recovery from whatever disease was occurring. Cayenne is not irritating when uncooked.

Cayenne powder or tincture can be rubbed on toothaches, swellings and inflammations. A remedy for arthritis is to rub a little cayenne tincture over the inflamed joint and wrap a red flannel around it to remain throughout the night. The pain is usually relieved by morning.

For hemorrhage internally or externally, cayenne can be relied on to stop the bleeding by virtue of the fact that it normalizes the circulation. For the same reason, it is very well suited for those who have either high or low blood pressure.

When a little cayenne is combined with plantain and applied as a poultice, it has remarkable powers to draw out any foreign object embedded in the flesh.

Cinnamon *(Cinnamomum zeylanicum)*

Cinnamon is stimulating, astringent, demulcent and carminative. It warms the system and is useful to add to balance cooling foods such as fruits, milk and desserts. Medicinally it is used to warm the organs to treat chronic diarrhea, cramps, heart and abdominal pains, coughing, wheezing and lower back pain. It is effectively used as a tincture given every fifteen minutes or so to stop bleeding from the uterus. Simmered in milk and taken with a little honey, cinnamon is very effective for indigestion, gas, diarrhea and dysentery.

Cloves *(Eugenia aromatica)*

Cloves are stimulating aromatic buds of the clove tree and are effective in warming the body, increasing circulation, improving digestion and treating flatulence, vomiting and nausea. They will also help the action of other medicines. Allspice *(Pimenta officinalis)* has a very similar action and may be substituted. Add cloves or allspice to any herbal formula requiring a stimulant (see the chapter on "Making an Herbal Formula"). Oil of cloves gives quick relief for toothaches, and cloves may simply be chewed for this purpose.

Coriander *(Coriandrum sativum)*

The coriander seeds are added to hot stimulating foods to impart a balanced coolness. It is diuretic, alterative and carminative. Steeped in tea, it is useful to relieve fevers (a small amount of black pepper may be added to stimulate its action). Use two teaspoons of crushed seeds in a cup of boiled water and steep twenty minutes. Coriander is added to laxative formulas to help prevent griping.

Cumin *(Cuminum cyminum)*

Cumin is an essential ingredient in making curries. It is one of the best spices to use to prevent and relieve gas (carminative). As such it is particularly useful to cook beans and fried foods with cumin. It is also a stimulant and antispasmodic useful in formulas calling for both qualities (see the chapter on "Making an Herbal Formula"). Cumin is of benefit to the heart and uterus and is given to women after childbirth to increase breast milk (galactogogue). The seeds may be used to make a tea (one teaspoon crushed seeds to a cup of boiled water) but because of the strong flavor, the powdered seeds may be taken in gelatin capsules, two capsules at mealtime in the evening. Externally, cumin can be used in liniments for stimulating circulation and bringing warmth to the area (see the "Methods of Application" chapter).

Fennel *(Foeniculum vulgare)*

Fennel is a very valuable seed spice combining several herbal properties. It is antispasmodic, carminative, diuretic, expectorant and stimulant. A tea is made using one teaspoon of crushed seeds in a cup of boiled water, steeped twenty minutes. This is used to treat colic, cramps and gas, and to expel mucus. The cooled tea can also be used externally as an eyewash. Fennel is useful in herb formulas containing strong laxatives to prevent griping. For chronic coughs, fennel may be used in making cough syrups (see the "Methods of Application" chapter).

Fenugreek *(Trigonella foenumgraecum)*

Fenugreek is one of the oldest recorded medicinal plants and one of the most versatile of the seed spices. The seeds are tonic, astringent, demulcent, emollient and expectorant. Fenugreek is useful for all mucous conditions and lung congestion. A decoction is made using one ounce of the crushed seeds with seven crushed black peppercorns in a pint of water to relieve congestion and eliminate excess mucus. The decoction of fenugreek alone is useful for ulcers and inflamed conditions of the stomach and intestines. It is also used in the treatment of both diabetes and gout. Fenugreek is considered to be an aphrodisiac and rejuvenator. Externally, it is used to make an emollient poultice applied to boils and carbuncles.

Garlic *(Allium sativum)*

Garlic is a world-renowned cure-all highly espoused as a home remedy in practically every culture. It has the properties of being an alterative, stimulant, diaphoretic, expectorant, antispasmodic, antibiotic, nervine, carminative and vulnerary, to mention some of the more outstanding characteristics.

It is used in the treatment of all lung ailments, for high and low blood pressure, against parasites and infections, for headaches and for nervous disorders. Onions have similar characteristics and are often used in combination with garlic.

To preserve the beneficial effects of garlic it should not be boiled. The fresh juice is the most effective preparation. For nervous spasms, cramps and seizures, crush one clove of garlic in a glass of hot milk. For high blood pressure, take one clove of garlic each morning.

Prepare oil of garlic by placing eight ounces of peeled minced garlic in a wide-mouthed jar with enough olive oil to cover. Close tightly and shake it a few times each day; allow it to stand in a warm place for three days. Press and strain it through an unbleached muslin or cotton cloth and store in a cool place.

For colds, flus, fevers and infectious diseases take one teaspoon of the oil every hour. For earaches, insert a few drops in the ear with a wad of cotton. For aches, sprains and minor skin disorders rub the oil directly on the affected area.

Prepare syrup of garlic by placing one pound of peeled minced garlic in a wide-mouthed two quart jar and almost fill the jar with equal parts of apple cider vinegar and distilled water. Cover and let stand in a warm place for four days, shaking a few times a day. Add one cup of glycerine and let it stand another day. Strain and, with pressure, filter the mixture through a muslin or linen cloth. Add one cup of honey and stir until thoroughly mixed. Store in a cool place.

For coughs, colds, sore throats, bronchial congestion, high or low blood pressure, heart weakness and nervous disorders, take one tablespoon of the syrup three times a day before meals.

Ginger *(Zingiberis officianalis)*

Ginger is one of the most versatile herbal stimulants. It is of great benefit to the stomach, intestines and circulation. Ginger may be taken alone or with other herbs to enhance their effectiveness. Ginger tea, made by grating one ounce of fresh ginger and simmering ten minutes in a pint of water, is used for indigestion, cramps and nausea. Taken with honey and lemon it is an excellent treatment for colds and flus and acts as a stimulating diaphoretic. Ginger root should always be added to meat dishes to help the intestines detoxify the meat.

Externally, ginger is applied as a fomentation for the treatment of pain, inflammations and stiff joints. Simmer five ounces of grated ginger root in two quarts of water for ten minutes. Strain and soak a cloth in the water to apply to the affected area. Keep changing the cloth to keep a constant warm temperature on the skin. The skin should become red as the circulation increases.

Squeeze out the juice of fresh grated ginger and combine with equal parts of olive or sesame oil to produce an oil that can be massaged into the skin for relief of muscle pain. The oil can also be applied to the head for dandruff and a few drops on a wad of cotton inserted into the ear is good for treating earaches.

In all formulas calling for ginger, either the fresh or the dried root may be used unless otherwise specified. The amount used, by weight, is the same.

Marjoram *(Origanum majorana)*

Marjoram is an antispasmodic, diaphoretic, carminative, tonic, expectorant, stimulant and emmenagogue. The tea, made with one-half ounce marjoram steeped in a pint of boiled water, is used for upset stomach, headache, colic and a variety of nervous complaints. It can be used for cramps and nausea associated with menstruation

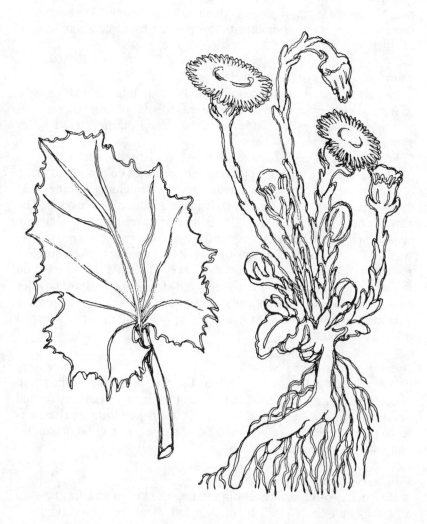

GINGER *(Zingiber officiale)*

The most versatile herbal stimulant for internal and external applications.

and for severe cases of abdominal cramps. It is also considered helpful for seasickness. Oil of marjoram can be used externally to relieve
aches and pains and can be applied for this purpose to toothaches. It
is added to the bath to promote a calming effect and to relieve insomnia. Marjoram is applied as a fomentation to painful swellings and
rheumatic joints and in liniments to stimulate the circulation (see the
chapter on "Methods of Application").

Mustard seed *(Brassica nigra)*

Mustard seed is rubefacient, stimulant, diuretic, alterative and,
in large doses, emetic. Internally, a teaspoonful of crushed seeds in
warm water acts as a mild laxative and blood purifier, but a table-
spoonful acts as a quick emetic.

Externally, the oil is used to stimulate local circulation. A mustard
plaster is made by mixing powdered mustard with cold water to make
a thick paste. The paste is spread on a cotton cloth. Another thin
cloth is placed on the skin and the mustard cloth placed over it. The
plaster should remain on until the skin begins to redden and a burning
sensation is felt. The plaster is removed and the remaining mustard is
washed from the skin. The mustard plaster is used for aches, sprains,
spasms and cold areas needing circulation. It should not be used on
tender, sensitive areas and if it seems too strong, the mustard powder
may be diluted with a little rye flour. After removing the plaster, the
skin may be powdered with rice or other flour and the area wrapped
with dry cotton.

Nutmeg *(Myristica fragans)*

A small amount of nutmeg, about the size of a pea, can be taken
once daily over a long period to relieve chronic nervous disorders and
heart problems. It may be added to milk and baked fruits and desserts
to help digestion and relieve nausea. Large doses can be poisonous
and may cause miscarriage.

Rosemary *(Rosmarinus officinalis)*

Rosemary is of great benefit in treating headaches and may be used
as a substitute for aspirin. It is astringent, diaphoretic and stimulant.
It is useful for indigestion, colic, nausea, gas and fevers. It is high in
easily assimilable calcium and thus is of benefit to the entire nervous
system. A tea is made by adding one-half ounce of rosemary to a pint
of boiled water and steeping for ten minutes in a covered vessel.
Rosemary is also good for the hair and scalp; use a cooled strong tea
as a rinse after shampoo. Rosemary is smoked with coltsfoot leaves
to treat asthma and mucous congestion of the lungs and throat.

Sage *(Salvia officinalis)*

Sage is antispasmodic and astringent and is of particular benefit in slowing the secretions of fluids. Thus it is used for excessive perspiration, night sweats, clear vaginal discharge and to stop the flow of milk. It is also useful for diarrhea, dysentery, the early stages of cold and flu, sinus congestion, bladder infections and inflammatory conditions. A tea is made using one-quarter ounce of the herb in a pint of boiled water, steeping in a closed vessel for ten minutes. It should not be used for more than one week at a time, but during this period the tea may be taken up to three times per day. When combined with rosemary, peppermint and wood betony, it is effective for headaches. A half cup of the infusion, made from equal parts of these herbs (one ounce per pint of water), is taken every two hours until relief is obtained. Sage tea is also used as a gargle for sore throats and ulcerations of the mouth.

Thyme *(Thymus vulgaris)*

Thyme is important as a parasiticide for intestinal worms. It is also antispasmodic, carminative, diaphoretic, expectorant and antiseptic. It is frequently used as a tea for bronchial problems such as acute bronchitis, whooping cough and laryngitis. An ounce of the herb is steeped in one pint of boiled water and then strained and sweetened with honey. It is also of benefit for the treatment of diarrhea, chronic gastritis and lack of appetite. It should not be used in large amounts, one ounce being adequate for a daily dose taken as tea. Externally, its antiseptic properties make it a useful mouthwash and cleansing wash for the skin. It will destroy fungal infections such as athlete's foot and skin parasites such as scabies, crabs and lice. For these purposes, a tincture made from four ounces thyme to a pint of alcohol, or the essential oil, is used.

Turmeric *(Curcuma longa)*

This root imparts its characteristic golden color to curry powder and to most Indian dishes. It is used as a blood purifier, stimulant and vulnerary. It can be applied both internally and externally to heal wounds, relieve pains in the limbs, break up congestion and as a restorative after the loss of blood at the birth of a child. It is of benefit to the circulation and it helps to regulate the menstrual cycle. Turmeric is also used for reducing fevers and for nosebleed. A teaspoon of turmeric powder is added along with a teaspoon of almond oil to a cup of warm milk. One to two cups are taken daily. This is particularly helpful in stretching the ligaments and to cure menstrual cramps.

9

HERBS TO KNOW

There are about half a million species of plants in the world. The modern Chinese pharmacopoeia, the most well-developed guide to medicinal plants, describes more than 10,000 plants that grow in China and are used for medicine. Even in areas with less well-developed herbal traditions, such as the United States, herbalists generally have a knowledge of about three hundred herbs. On the other hand, most herbalists make it their practice to utilize, in various combinations and by different methods of application, only about one hundred herbs for most situations.

In addition to the two dozen culinary herbs and spices that find their way into numerous herb formulas, there are about ninety other herbs that everyone interested in using herbal remedies should know. These are herbs that have the following characteristics:

1. they are very effective in the treatment of several ailments;
2. their properties have been well established by centuries of practical use;
3. they can be obtained almost anywhere, because they are commercially available;
4. they have a low toxicity so that they may be used safely when precautions are followed.

This chapter has been divided into two sections, one called "Western Herbs," referring to herbs primarily from outside the Orient, and one called "Chinese Herbs," including herbs that hold a special position in Chinese medicine. These Chinese herbs are sufficiently important to modern herbal practice that they should become generally known, but as yet, most of these are available primarily from shops in Chinatowns, either directly or by mail order.

It is interesting to note that a large number of the commonly used medicinal plants of the West come from three plant families:

Umbelliferae *(Apiaceae)*	*Compositae*	*Labiatae* *(Lamiaceae)*
Angelica	Blessed thistle	Catnip
Anise	Boneset	Hyssop
Caraway	Burdock	Lemon balm
Coriander	Calendula	Marjoram
Cumin	Chickory	Motherwort
Fennel	Coltsfoot	Pennyroyal (European)
Gota kola	Dandelion	Peppermint
Parsley	Dill	Rosemary
	Echinacea	Sage
	Elecampane	Skullcap
	Gravel root	Spearmint
	Mugwort	Stoneroot
	Wormwood	Thyme
	Yarrow	Wood betony

The reference to the part of the plant used is generally limited to that part available commercially. Often other parts of the plant are also used, but less commonly. If you gather the fresh herbs, it will be worthwhile to check on the uses of the other parts; some reference books are mentioned in the Bibliography. Frequently, one part of a plant will be a useful medicine, another part a useful food and another part a poison that must be avoided.

Properties of the herbs that are capitalized are the most important ones considered in making a formula and in finding substitutes. The other properties are of lesser importance, but are often valuable to know, for example, when the herb also acts as an emmenagogue in large quantities.

When not described in detail, the method of preparation of the herb is according to the instructions in the "Methods of Application" chapter. Dosages are calculated for a person weighing about 150 pounds (see the "Herbs for Children" section in the final chapter, "Cautionary Notes on Herb Use"); adjust the amount recommended to match the size of the person being treated.

Western Herbs

Agrimony   *Agrimonia eupatoria*
                                                   Rosaceae

PART USED: Aboveground portion
SYSTEMS AFFECTED: Stomach, intestines and liver
PROPERTIES: Hepatic tonic
                  Diuretic
                  Astringent
                  Vulnerary
                  antipyretic

Agrimony was used by the native American as a tonic to strengthen the whole system. It is specifically used for all digestive disorders and for strengthening the stomach, intestines, liver, gallbladder and kidneys. It is also good for treating inflammatory diseases and skin eruptions.

Externally, it can be applied for athlete's foot and to promote the healing of wounds and sores. It can be applied to treat venomous bites and stings and may also be taken internally for that purpose. A tincture is applied to the skin to draw out thorns and splinters. Agrimony is used in vaginal douches for treating abnormal discharges.

Agrimony should not be used when there is a dryness of the body secretions.

Gentian root (*Gentiana* spp.) is used like agrimony as a bitter tonic to stimulate the digestive organs. For internal use, both agrimony and gentian are prepared either as a tea, using one ounce to a pint of water, or as a tincture, using four ounces to a pint of alcohol. Agrimony is quite bitter and contains about 5% tannins, contributing to its astringency.

Alfalfa   *Medicago sativa*
                                         Leguminosae

PART USED: Leaves and flowers
SYSTEMS AFFECTED: Stomach and blood
PROPERTIES: Nutritive tonic
                  Antipyretic
                  Alterative

Alfalfa is used to help the assimilation of protein, calcium and other nutrients. Its cooling property makes it useful in reducing fevers. Alfalfa is very beneficial to the blood, acting as a blood purifier, as a remedy for anemia and to help stop bleeding. Red clover blossoms have similar properties and may be used as a substitute.

The fresh alfalfa leaves can be eaten in soups, salads or as a steamed vegetable. A beverage tea can be made using one or two teaspoons dried alfalfa per cup of water. The regular use of alfalfa will help normalize body weight, but, according to the Chinese, excessive use will cause one to lose weight and become thin.

Alfalfa is commonly added to other herbs for its nutritive qualities. It may be added as 10–20% of the formula.

Aloe vera

Aloe vera
Liliaceae

PART USED: Leaves
SYSTEMS AFFECTED: Skin, colon and stomach
PROPERTIES: Vulnerary
Laxative
Demulcent
Emollient
emmenagogue

The gel of the leaves of the aloe is most widely honored for its capacity to heal even the most severe burns and irritated skin rashes. In addition, it has been successfully applied for the treatment of insect bites and stings, poison oak and ivy, "detergent hands," acne and itchy skin.

Taken internally, it is a laxative and regulator of the bowels. Since its use alone might cause griping (cramping of the bowels), it is best to combine aloe with ginger root. This is also highly effective for treating ulcers. Combine four parts aloe powder with one part ginger root powder and fill "00" gelatin capsules. Take two capsules, three times a day. Alternatively one may take the bitter aloe gel in small quantities at regular intervals (totaling a pint a day for ulcers), along with a tea of ginger and licorice root to help prevent any adverse reactions to the bitter taste.

Aloe plants are readily obtained, and they grow well in the home. As a first aid remedy for burns and irritations, break off a leaf and squeeze the gel onto the affected area.

Amaranth

Amaranthus spp.
Americanaceae

PART USED: Leaves and flowers
SYSTEMS AFFECTED: Blood, genitourinary tract, stomach
and spleen
PROPERTIES: Astringent
Hemostatic
Diuretic
alterative

Amaranth is a highly effective treatment for bleeding, used especially for excessive menstruation, but also for all internal and external wounds. Its astringent properties also make it an excellent treatment for diarrhea and dysentery.

The leaves are used much like spinach. Amaranth is a common garden weed, readily available fresh. The dried leaves and flowers are taken internally as a decoction using a pint of water to an ounce of herb and simmering in a closed vessel. A half cup is taken each time, as needed to stop bleeding or to check diarrhea. Either the tincture or the decoction is applied externally to sores and ulcerated conditions. The decoction is used in a douche for leukorrhea (whites).

Angelica   *Angelica archangelica*
                                                         Umbelliferae

PART USED: Root
SYSTEMS AFFECTED: Circulation, heart, lungs, skin, stomach
                    and intestines
PROPERTIES: Stimulant
            Tonic
            Emmenagogue
            Carminative
            diaphoretic
            expectorant
            alterative

Angelica is used to improve the circulation and warm the body. It is one of the best herbs to use for coldness in the winter. Because of its warming properties, it relieves spasms of the stomach and intestines and dispels gas. Its regular use will create a distaste for alcoholic drinks.

Angelica is a strong emmenagogue and should not be used by pregnant women. It should not be used by diabetics, as it tends to increase the sugar in the blood.

Angelica is of great benefit in the treatment of colds, coughs, pleurisy and all lung diseases. It is also used in the treatment of rheumatism, especially applied externally as a poultice or liniment.

The tea is prepared as an infusion, with a pint of boiled water poured over an ounce of the bruised root. The usual dose is two or three tablespoons, three times daily. The powdered root may be taken in gelatin capsules, two capsules each time. A tincture made with four ounces of the root per pint of alcohol is taken one teaspoon each time.

Bayberry   *Myrica cerifera*
                                                                Myricaceae

PART USED: Bark
SYSTEMS AFFECTED: Skin, circulation, stomach and intestines
PROPERTIES: Astringent
            Stimulant

The most renowned use of bayberry bark is as the prime ingredient in "Dr. Thompson's Composition Powder." This powder is a tonic, stimulating medicine that raises vitality and resistance to disease. There are several variations of composition powder, but they all combine bayberry bark with a number of other herbal stimulants (see the "Making an Herbal Formula" chapter).

Bayberry is useful wherever an astringent is required. If not available, white oak bark may be substituted, although it does not have the stimulating properties of the bayberry bark.

This potent herb can be made into a tea using one teaspoon to a cup of hot water. Taken as a warm infusion, bayberry will induce perspiration, improve circulation and tone all the tissues it contacts. In large doses, it acts as an emetic. It may be used as a gargle for sore throat. A fomentation made from this tea can be applied externally at night to relieve, cure and prevent varicose veins.

Bayberry bark is used to treat prolapsed uterus and excessive menstrual bleeding, and may be used in a douche to treat vaginal discharge. It has also been valued for stopping hemorrhage of the bowels, lungs and uterus. The powder may be taken in gelatin capsules, two at a time as needed. Direct application of the powder to the gums is good for managing pyorrhea.

Be careful not to confuse bayberry bark with barberry bark (*Berberis vulgaris*). Barberry bark is a hepatic tonic, laxative and antiseptic. It is an excellent treatment for poor digestion and has properties similar to Oregon grape root.

Blackberry   *Rubus villosus*
                                                                Rosaceae

PART USED: Leaves and root bark
SYSTEMS AFFECTED: Colon and blood
PROPERTIES: Astringent
            Hemostatic
            diuretic

There is perhaps no better remedy for diarrhea, dysentery and bleeding than that of blackberry root bark. Simmer a tablespoon of the root bark with one teaspoon of cinnamon powder in one cup of milk for five minutes on low heat. This may be taken with a little honey, or more effectively without a sweetener. The combination of blackberry and cinnamon is also effective if boiled for twenty minutes in one and one-half cups of water. One-half cup is taken four times daily until relief is obtained.

For milder cases of diarrhea, fevers or sore throats one can use a decoction of either one, or a combination, of the leaves, buds and branches of the blackberry bush, using one ounce of herb to a pint of water (simmer at least fifteen minutes, covered). Take one-half cup, four times a day. The tea may be sweetened if desired.

Black cohosh

Cimicifuga racemosa
Ranunculaceae

PART USED: Root
SYSTEMS AFFECTED: Uterus, nerves, lungs and heart
PROPERTIES: Antispasmodic
          Alterative
          Emmenagogue
          diuretic

Black cohosh is a useful antispasmodic for all nervous conditions, cramps and pains. Native American women used black cohosh to relieve the pains associated with childbirth and with the menstrual cycle. It has been used for neuralgia, hysteria and bronchial spasms. Combined in a tincture or in capsules with equal parts of elecampane and wild cherry bark, and taken with a tea of yerba santa, it is an excellent remedy for whooping cough, asthma and bronchitis.

Black cohosh has also been used for eruptive diseases, such as measles, and for rheumatism. It is an excellent remedy for high blood pressure.

The average dosage is one "00" capsule or fifteen to thirty drops of the tincture taken six times a day. Too large a dose will cause nausea and dizziness.

Blessed thistle

Cerbenia benedicta
Compositae

PART USED: Aboveground portion
SYSTEMS AFFECTED: Stomach, heart, blood, mammary glands
                 and uterus

PROPERTIES: Tonic
Galactogogue
Emmenagogue
Stimulant
Alterative
Diaphoretic
emetic

Blessed thistle is an excellent stimulant tonic for the stomach and heart. It aids circulation and helps resolve all liver problems.

It is well noted for increasing mother's milk, especially when taken with equal parts raspberry leaves and marshmallow root. Blessed thistle is used in many formulas for treating painful menstruation.

An infusion is made using one ounce of the herb to a pint of boiled water. It is taken one-half cup each time, three times daily between meals. Alternatively, the tincture is made and taken in doses of one tablespoon each time. If taken in excess, it will act as an emetic.

Blue cohosh   *Caulophyllum thalictroides*
                                     Berberidaceae

PART USED: Root
SYSTEMS AFFECTED: Uterus, nerves, joints and urinary tract
PROPERTIES: Oxytocic
Antispasmodic
Emmenagogue
Diuretic

Blue cohosh was widely used among the native Americans to relieve menstrual cramps and the pains associated with childbirth. It was taken during the last month of pregnancy to aid in a speedy and painless delivery. Because of its emmenagogue properties, it is not to be used by pregnant women except during the last month of pregnancy.

Blue cohosh is often combined with black cohosh because the herbs have complementary properties beneficial for the nerves and a strong antispasmodic effect on the entire system. It is combined with other herbs to promote their effects in treating bronchitis, nervous disorders, urinary tract ailments and rheumatism.

Prepare a tincture of blue cohosh or a combination of both blue and black cohoshes, using four ounces of root powder per pint of alcohol. Standard dose is fifteen to thirty drops, three times daily. Alternatively, one may fill gelatin capsules and take one at a time. Neither blue cohosh nor black cohosh is used in teas because some of the active principles are not soluble in water.

Boneset   *Eupatorium perfoliatum*
                                               Compositae

PART USED: Aboveground portion
SYSTEMS AFFECTED: Stomach, liver, intestines, uterus
                        and circulation
PROPERTIES: Stimulant
             Antipyretic
             Diaphoretic
             Laxative

Boneset is particularly useful for treating fevers, especially inter-
mittent fevers. It is widely used for flus and catarrh, taken as a warm
infusion. The tea is made using an ounce of herb to a pint of water,
steeped ten minutes. One-half cup is taken three times daily. When it
is taken cold it is a tonic stimulant. The hot tea is used for sweating
therapy, using four or five half-cup doses while in bed.

Boneset is a very bitter herb that stimulates digestion and elimination. It should be taken without sweetening, except for treating
coughs and catarrh. The tincture may be used, taking one to two
tablespoons at a time.

Borage   *Borago officinalis*
                                               Boraginaceae

PART USED: Leaves
SYSTEMS AFFECTED: Circulation, kidneys, lungs and skin
PROPERTIES: Antipyretic
             Diuretic
             Emollient
             galactogogue

Borage is a valuable remedy for reducing high fevers. It is taken
as a tea for all lung problems, especially chronic catarrh. It is strengthening to the heart. Make an infusion using one ounce of herb to a pint
of water. Take one-half cup three times daily.

Externally, borage is used for all irritations of the skin and mucous
membranes. It may be applied as the tincture or can be used as an
ingredient in salves and liniments.

Buchu   *Barosma betulina*
                                               Rutaceae

PART USED: Leaves
SYSTEMS AFFECTED: Kidneys and bladder
PROPERTIES: Diuretic
             Antiseptic
             Diaphoretic

Buchu leaves are one of the best diuretics known. The herb is used for all acute and chronic bladder and kidney disorders, including inflammation of the urethra, nephritis, cystitis and catarrh of the bladder.

As with most diuretics, buchu works better if it is given as a cool infusion. Buchu is commonly combined with uva ursi for the treatment of water retention and urinary tract infections. Do not boil buchu or uva ursi, as their active principles are volatile oils.

When given warm it is a stimulating diaphoretic useful in the treatment of enlargement of the prostrate gland and irritation of the membrane of the urethra. Make an infusion using one ounce of buchu leaves to a pint of water. For an after dinner beverage tea to replace coffee, combine:

> Buchu leaves — 2 parts
> Uva ursi — 2 parts
> Orange peel — 1 part
> Peppermint — 1 part
> Camomile — 1 part
> Comfrey leaves — 1 part

Use one-quarter ounce of the herb mixture in a pint of boiled water and steep for ten minutes. This will also strengthen the kidneys.

Burdock   *Arctium lappa*
                                                         Compositae

PART USED: Root
SYSTEMS AFFECTED: Blood and kidneys; general effects on
                 the whole body
PROPERTIES: Alterative
            Diuretic
            Diaphoretic
            Tonic
            Demulcent

Burdock contains 27–45% inulin, the source of most of its curative powers. Inulin, commonly found in plants of the *Compositae* family, such as dandelion, is a form of starch. Burdock also provides an abundance of iron, which makes it of special value for the blood. It is also a valuable blood purifier and is used in this capacity for the treatment of arthritis, rheumatism, sciatica and lumbago.

Burdock is used to promote kidney function and works through the kidneys to help clear the blood of harmful acids.

The diaphoretic property of burdock is due to the presence of a volatile oil, which, when taken internally, is eliminated from the sweat glands, thus removing toxic wastes. Sweating has a cooling effect on the body; burdock is therefore used to clear fevers and heat conditions (Yang diseases) such as boils, styes, carbuncles, canker sores and infections.

The Chinese use burdock to eliminate excess nervous energy and also consider it to be a strengthening aphrodisiac.

Burdock is an excellent remedy for all skin diseases, taken alone or with other blood purifiers such as sarsaparilla. Make a decoction of the root using one ounce to one and one-half pints of water and simmer until the volume is reduced to one pint. Take one-half cup, three times daily. For sweating, simmer covered for ten minutes and drink one cup of the tea before taking a hot bath.

Calamus   *Acorus calamus*
Araceae

PART USED: Rhizome
SYSTEMS AFFECTED: Stomach, intestines and liver
PROPERTIES: Stomach tonic
             Antispasmodic

Calamus is an invaluable remedy for hyperacidity associated with the stomach and intestines. It has a beneficial effect on the liver and can be used to treat most diseases of the stomach, intestines and liver.

Calamus is a useful aid to quitting smoking, since if one chews the dried root and afterwards tries to smoke, a mild nausea will result, which will discourage the habit. The Northwestern Indians, when running long distances, would keep a piece in the mouth to increase endurance and stamina.

Externally, it is added to the bath to quiet the nerves and induce a tranquil state. The tincture is useful as a parasiticide applied at regular intervals to the skin in the treatment of scabies, lice or crabs.

Calamus is taken internally only in small amounts. Usually, one chews a small amount of it, or the powder may be used in gelatin capsules, only one capsule taken each time it is needed.

Calendula   *Calendula officinalis*
Compositae

PART USED: Flowers
SYSTEMS AFFECTED: Blood and skin
PROPERTIES: Vulnerary
             Astringent
             Diaphoretic
             antispasmodic

Calendula, used as an oil, in a salve or as a poultice will stop bleeding, soothe pain and irritation and promote mending and healing of wounds. It is used internally as a warm infusion to treat fevers, ulcers, cramps and eruptive skin diseases.

The tea, made with one ounce of herb per pint of water, may be taken hourly for acute ailments. The oil can be placed in the ears with

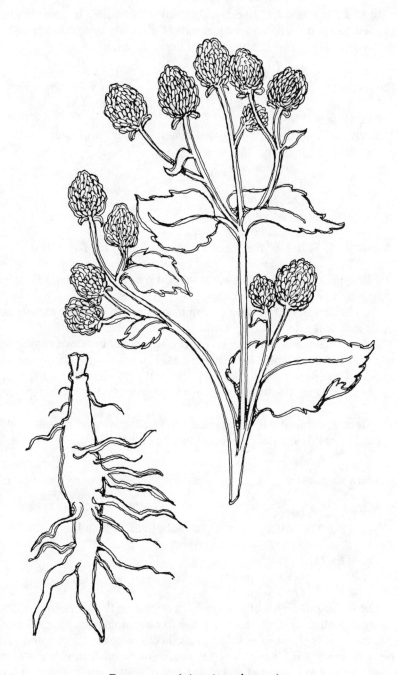

BURDOCK (*Arctium lappa*)

An excellent remedy for all skin diseases.

a bit of cotton and left overnight to relieve earache. It may also be applied to treat bleeding hemorrhoids. Calendula is commonly used in making salves and is a very good first aid remedy.

Camomile   *Matricaria chamomilla*
                                                Compositae

PART USED: Flower
SYSTEMS AFFECTED: Nerves, stomach, kidneys and liver
PROPERTIES: Nervine
                Carminative
                Tonic
                Diaphoretic
                Sedative
                emmenagogue

Camomile is one of the most widely used beverage and medicinal teas. It is a valuable calming drink for restlessness, nervous stomach and insomnia. It is safely used for children in the treatment of colds, indigestion and nervous disorders.

Camomile will help relieve cramping associated with the menstrual cycle and will bring on the period.

A beverage tea is made by steeping one-quarter ounce of camomile in a pint of boiled water for ten minutes. For a stronger effect, use an ounce of the flowers to a pint of water and drink one-half cup of the tea as needed. A tincture is also used, taken one to two tablespoons at a time.

Externally, camomile is applied to swellings, sore muscles and painful joints. It is also frequently used as a hair rinse.

Cascara sagrada   *Rhamnus purshiana*
                                                Rhamnaceae

PART USED: Bark
SYSTEMS AFFECTED: Colon, stomach, liver, gallbladder
                        and pancreas
PROPERTIES: Laxative
                Hepatic tonic
                antispasmodic

The bitter principles of cascara bark stimulate the secretions of the entire digestive system, including the liver, gallbladder, stomach and pancreas. It is one of the safest tonic-laxative herbs known and can be used on a daily basis without becoming habit-forming. Cascara is very valuable whenever there are hemorrhoids associated with poor bowel function. The tincture can be used for a gentle laxative, using twenty to twenty-five drops, three times a day. For faster action, increase the dose, using from one-half to three-quarters of a teaspoon of the tincture. (See Dr. Christopher's lower bowel tonic in the chapter on "Making an Herbal Formula.") To prevent griping, anise, caraway or fennel seeds may be taken at the same time as the cascara when it is used as a laxative. Cascara is generally not taken as a tea.

Catnip   *Nepata cataria*
                                                              Labiatae

PART USED: Aboveground portion
SYSTEMS AFFECTED: Nerves and intestines
PROPERTIES: Diaphoretic
            Sedative
            Nervine
            Carminative

Catnip is famous for its sedative effects on the nervous system. It gently relieves the "congestion" affecting the nerves as a result of built-up emotional tensions.

Catnip is a good cure for diarrhea and is frequently used in enemas to relax and gently restore the tone of the bowels. It is an excellent herb for children, especially when mixed in a tea with camomile, spearmint and lemon balm.

Catnip tea is made using one ounce of herb per pint of water, steeped twenty minutes. It is useful in formulas for insomnia. Catnip has been smoked for its calming effects, but it may cause headaches when taken that way.

Chaparral   *Larrea divaricata*
                                                              Zygophyllaceae

PART USED: Leaves and stems
SYSTEMS AFFECTED: Stomach, intestines and lungs; general
                 effects on whole body
PROPERTIES: Antiseptic
            Antibiotic
            Parasiticide
            Alterative
            expectorant
            diuretic

Chaparral is one of the best herbal antibiotics, being useful against bacteria, viruses and parasites, both internally and externally. It may be taken internally for colds and flus, inflammations of the respiratory tract and intestinal tract, diarrhea and urinary tract infections.

Chaparral is usually taken as a tincture, one teaspoon per dose, or in capsules or pills, two per dose. It is frequently combined with other antibiotic herbs such as goldenseal and echinacea.

Externally, chaparral is applied to wounds as an antiseptic, to the skin in the treatment of itching, eczema and scabies and to the scalp as a hair tonic and for dandruff. A liniment made from chaparral or a bath made by soaking the leaves in the water is used for rheumatism. A concentrate of the extract can be applied to warts to reduce them.

Chaparral contains a substance called NDGA, which is a powerful antioxidant, useful in preserving fats and oils, and an anti-tumor agent. The native Americans used it to treat cancer.

Chickweed   *Stellaria media*
                                                      Caryophyllaceae

PART USED: Aboveground portion
SYSTEMS AFFECTED: Blood, liver, lungs, kidneys and bladder
PROPERTIES: Demulcent
            Alterative
            Antipyretic

Chickweed is a common wayside weed with great value in treating blood toxicity, fevers, inflammation and other characteristically "hot" diseases. It is a mild herb used as food as well as medicine; therefore it is considered to be as safe as most vegetables and can be used in high dosage whenever needed.

Chickweed tea is prepared as a decoction, using an ounce of herb simmered in a pint of water for thirty minutes. Use one-half cup, three times daily. The tincture may also be used, taken in doses of one tablespoon.

Chickweed is particularly useful for reducing excess fat, having both mild diuretic and laxative properties. Externally it is used in the form of a poultice applied directly to boils and abscesses. It is also made into an oil and ointment and used for a wide variety of sores and other cutaneous diseases.

Cleavers   *Galium aparine*
                                                      Rubiaceae

PART USED: Aboveground portion
SYSTEMS AFFECTED: Kidneys, bladder, blood and skin
PROPERTIES: Diuretic
            Astringent
            Laxative
            Antipyretic
            Alterative

Cleavers is highly recommended for all kidney and bladder problems, especially obstructions of the urinary organs, such as stones and gravel. It is a powerful diuretic useful in reducing weight and treating edema. It is often combined with equal parts uva ursi and buchu and one-quarter part each of marshmallow and ginger.

Cleavers, taken internally, is also valuable for treating skin diseases and eruptions. Externally it is used in a salve for scalds and burns. Its cooling properties make it a good treatment for fevers.

A tea is made by infusing one ounce of cleavers in a pint of water. A tincture is also a valuable way of taking cleavers, one teaspoon taken three times daily.

Coltsfoot   *Tussilago farfara*
                                                      Compositae

PART USED: Leaves
SYSTEMS AFFECTED: Lungs
PROPERTIES: Expectorant
            Emollient
            Demulcent

Tussilago means cough dispeller. Coltsfoot is one of the best cough remedies and may be smoked for relief of asthma, bronchitis and difficulty in breathing. For these purposes it can also be taken as a tea, especially in combination with horehound and marshmallow. It is also used in the treatment of swellings and inflammations. Make an infusion using one ounce of coltsfoot in a pint of boiled water. Take one-half cup, three times daily.

Comfrey   *Symphytum officinale*
                                                    Boraginaceae

PART USED: Leaves and roots
SYSTEMS AFFECTED: Bones and muscles; general effects on the
                 whole body
PROPERTIES: Demulcent
            Vulnerary
            Expectorant
            nutritive tonic
            alterative
            astringent

Comfrey has a healing and soothing effect upon every organ it contacts. It may be used both internally and externally for healing of fractures, wounds, sores and ulcers. Comfrey aids cell proliferation, thus helping to heal wounds rapidly. It is of great value to check hemorrhage, whether it be from the stomach, lungs, bowels, kidneys or piles. For bleeding, use a strong decoction of the root, using one-half to one ounce of root every two hours until the bleeding has stopped.

Comfrey will help the pancreas in regulating blood sugar levels. It helps relieve irritations associated with the gallbladder, kidneys, bladder, small intestines and stomach. It helps promote the secretion of pepsin and is a general aid to the digestion.

Its demulcent properties, especially of the root, have been used to treat lung troubles and coughs. Comfrey root has the highest content of mucilage of any of the herbs.

Comfrey is extremely prolific and versatile. A small piece of the root will reproduce itself in any shady moist area in a very short time.

A common addition to herb formulas, especially for the treatment of lung ailments, is comfrey mucilage. Soak two ounces of dried comfrey root in one quart of water overnight. Simmer in a covered container for thirty minutes, strain, filter and squeeze through a muslin or linen cloth. Return the extract to the cleaned vessel and add six ounces of honey and two ounces of glycerine, and simmer for five minutes. Cool and store in a wide-mouthed bottle. Take two tablespoons every hour for acute diseases (including internal hemorrhage) or three to four times daily for chronic ailments.

Cramp bark   *Viburnum opulis*
                                                              Caprifoliaceae

PART USED: Bark
SYSTEMS AFFECTED: Nerves, heart and genitourinary organs
PROPERTIES: Antispasmodic
                  Astringent
                  Nervine

Cramp bark is of great benefit for the relief of menstrual cramps. It can be combined with equal parts of ginger and angelica root and three parts camomile, and taken as a warm tea for all cramps and convulsions. It is also useful for the acute treatment of heart palpitation and rheumatism. Cramp bark can be used in the treatment of asthma. The decoction is made using one-half ounce of the bark in a pint of water. The dose is one tablespoon, taken frequently, as needed. A tincture made with four ounces of the bark in a pint of alcohol is taken one teaspoon per dose.

Cramp bark has properties very similar to black haw (*Viburnum prunifolium*) and this may be substituted when available.

Dandelion   *Taraxacum officinale*
                                          Compositae

PART USED: Leaves and roots
SYSTEMS AFFECTED: Liver, kidneys, gallbladder, pancreas
                  and blood
PROPERTIES: Hepatic tonic
            Diuretic
            Stomachic
            Lithotriptic
            astringent
            cholagogue
            galactogogue

The chief benefits of this great herb are exerted upon the function of the liver, and it has the capacity to clear obstructions and stimulate the liver to detoxify poisons. Thus dandelion serves as a blood purifier. Much of its beneficial action upon the liver and the blood is a result of its high content of easily assimilable minerals, especially in the root.

Dandelion root is also useful for clearing obstructions of the spleen, pancreas, gallbladder, bladder and kidneys. It is of tremendous benefit to the stomach and intestines. To treat stomachaches, drink one-half cup of the infusion every half hour until relief is attained.

Serious cases of hepatitis have been cured with the use of dandelion root tea within a week or two when the diet is controlled properly and limited to easily-digested foods (see remarks on "Therapeutic Diet" in the "Kitchen Medicines" chapter).

I consider dandelion root a specific for hypoglycemia. A cup of dandelion tea should be taken two or three times a day and the balanced diet (see the chapter on "A Balanced Diet") must be followed. Similarly, with a good diet, dandelion root tea can cure diabetes that has been acquired later in one's life.

Dandelion root is also of benefit in helping to lower blood pressure, thus aiding the action of the heart. It can also be helpful in treating anemia by supplying the necessary nutritive minerals.

The young dandelion leaves can be eaten fresh to obtain an abundance of vitamins and minerals that will be of great value to the nerves and the blood.

Chicory (*Cichorium endiva*) has properties very similar to dandelion and the two are commonly combined in making the medicinal tea and as a substitute for coffee. The roasted roots are used to produce a flavor like coffee, but the raw should be used in making a medicinal tea, with a small amount of the roasted roots added for flavor.

Echinacea   *Echinacea angustifolia,*
                                           Echinacea purpurea
                                           Compositae

PART USED: Root
SYSTEMS AFFECTED: Blood and lymph
PROPERTIES: Alterative
            Paraciticide
            Antiseptic
            Sialagogue
            Analgesic

Echinacea is the king of the blood purifiers. It is the most effective blood and lymphatic cleanser in the botanical kingdom. It can be used both internally and externally. Echinacea is a valuable alternative to all antibiotics when used properly.

The only times I have ever found echinacea ineffective have been when not enough has been taken. The amazing thing about this plant is that it is apparently nontoxic. In some it may cause mild dizziness or nausea for a time, but I have found that combining it with a small amount of licorice root or making the tea with two or three dates will ameliorate those symptoms.

Echinacea is useful for treating gangrene, blood poisoning and all chronic and acute bacterial and viral infections. It is effective against all venomous bites from insects, snakes and other animals, and against reactions to poison oak and poison ivy. Echinacea has a long history of use against syphilis and gonorrhea and is used in douches for the treatment of all vaginal infections.

For acute ailments it must be taken every hour ot two, as a tincture (one teaspoon) or a powder in two "00" capsules.

Elder   *Sambucus nigra*
                                           Caprifoliaceae

PART USED: Flowers
SYSTEMS AFFECTED: Blood, circulation, lungs, bowels and skin
PROPERTIES: Diaphoretic
            Alterative
            laxative
            stimulant

The elder flowers are used in the first stages of colds and flus. Combine equal parts of elder flowers and peppermint to make a tea (one ounce of herb per pint of water) and drink as hot as possible. Take the tea in bed, or just before taking a hot bath, and then sweat out the cold or flu during sleep.

Elder flowers are also used in salves for the treatment of burns, rashes and minor skin ailments. Other parts of the elder tree are used medicinally, but they may cause a toxic reaction. However, the bark and leaves can also be used in making a salve.

Elecampane
Inula helinum
Compositae

PART USED: Root
SYSTEMS AFFECTED: Lungs, stomach and spleen
PROPERTIES: Expectorant
Stimulant
Stomach tonic
diuretic
cholagogue
astringent

Elecampane is considered to be of great benefit for colic, cough and bronchitis, for which an ounce of the root is bruised and then extracted in a pint of red wine. For chronic lung ailments, combine with wild cherry bark, white pine bark, comfrey root and licorice. It is an excellent treatment for catarrh.

It is also very useful for digestive disorders, including weak digestion in the stomach and poor assimilation. The Chinese use it to counteract ingested poisons. A decoction is made using an ounce of the root, simmered in a pint of water for one hour. It is taken in doses of two teaspoons as needed. The powdered root is taken in capsules, one capsule, three times daily, or take one-half teaspoon of the tincture for each dose.

Eyebright
Euphrasia officinalis
Scrophularaceae

PART USED: Aboveground portion
SYSTEMS AFFECTED: Eyes, liver and blood
PROPERTIES: Alterative
Astringent
Tonic

Eyebright has a cooling and detoxifying property that makes it especially useful for inflammations. It aids in stimulating the liver to clear the blood and relieve those conditions that affect the clarity of vision and thought. The tea should be taken liberally and on a daily basis to treat all eye problems. It is also useful with inflammations of the nose and throat.

Externally, the tea is used as an eyewash, especially combined with goldenseal, rue or fennel, for conjunctivitis, eye weakness, opthalmia and other eye diseases.

The infusion is made using one ounce of herb to a pint of boiled water, steeped twenty minutes. A beverage tea useful as a substitute for black tea is prepared using one-half ounce of herb steeped in a pint of water.

False unicorn

Chamailirium luteum
Liliaceae

PART USED: Root
SYSTEMS AFFECTED: Uterus and kidneys
PROPERTIES: Uterine tonic
      Diuretic
      stimulant
      parasiticide
      emetic

The most common use of this herb is in the treatment of female sterility and impotence. Herbalists caution that if a woman does not want to get pregnant, she should not take any false unicorn root. To strengthen female fertility and prevent miscarriage, false unicorn may be taken daily for several months. One or two "00" gelatin capsules of the powdered root are taken three times daily, alone or in combination with other herbs.

The root is also used in the treatment of amenorrhea, painful menstruation, irregular menstruation and leukorrhea. It may be taken in small amounts during the early part of pregnancy to relieve morning sickness.

The true unicorn root, also known as star grass *(Aletris farinosa)* has similar properties and may be substituted.

Goldenseal

Hydrastis canadensis
Ranunculaceae

PART USED: Rhizome and root
SYSTEMS AFFECTED: Stomach, intestines, spleen, liver, eyes and
                all mucous membranes
PROPERTIES: Tonic
      Stimulant
      Antiseptic
      Alterative
      laxative
      emmenagogue

It is difficult to find a disease for which goldenseal would not be useful. Taken with any herb, it increases the tonic properties for the specific organs that are being treated. It is thus used with eyebright as a tonic for the eyes; with gota kola as a tonic for the brain; with

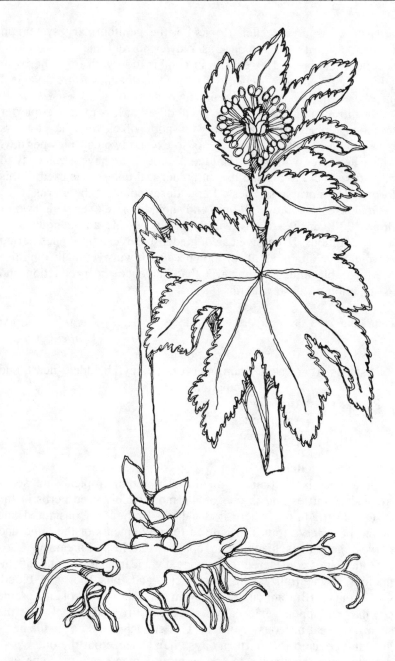

GOLDENSEAL (*Hydrastis canadensis*)

Useful in the treatment of almost every disease.
Externally applied in salves to prevent and fight infection.

squawvine as an excellent tonic for the genitourinary system in women; and with cascara bark as a lower bowel tonic.

Goldenseal is used externally in combination with other herbs in salves for its antiseptic effect. It is used in douches to treat vaginal infections and is effective in reducing hemorrhoids.

For morning sickness, use in small doses of less than one-quarter teaspoon along with one-quarter teaspoon of cloves, the powders being taken in gelatin capsules, not to exceed two capsules per day. These are taken with spearmint tea. Women who have a tendency to miscarry should avoid the use of goldenseal unless it is used in this formula for morning sickness. Large doses contract the uterus.

Goldenseal is a powerful herb and should not be overused. Two or three "00" capsules a day will generally be safe and adequate for most conditions. Excessive use of goldenseal over a prolonged period can diminish Vitamin B absorption because it will eventually diminish the favorable intestinal bacteria that influence the production and assimilation of these vitamins.

Gota kola   *Centella asiatica*
                                               Umbelliferae

PART USED: Aboveground portion
SYSTEMS AFFECTED: Brain, nerves, kidney, bladder, heart and
                 circulation
PROPERTIES: Alterative
            Antipyretic
            Brain tonic
            nervine
            diuretic

Gota kola is a common medicinal plant in tropical and semi-tropical countries and is one of the most widely used herbs in the Ayurvedic tradition (where it is called "Brahmi"). Considered one of the best nerve tonics, it is used for all ailments of the mind and nerves, including schizophrenia, epilepsy and loss of memory.

Gota kola is considered to be of great value in all fevers and inflammations. It neutralizes the blood acids and thus cools the blood. Gota kola oil (Brahmi oil), made by an extract of gota kola in sesame oil, may be applied externally over the entire body—including the scalp—to treat nervous disorders. Use enough oil to cover the herb, let stand covered for fourteen days, then squeeze out the oil.

Gota kola was known to Indian writers many centuries ago as a plant to increase longevity. It is taken as a tea, using an ounce of the herb per pint of water. One-half cup of tea is taken three times daily for at least one month.

Gravel Root *Eupatorium purpureum*
Compositae

PART USED: Root
SYSTEMS AFFECTED: Kidneys, bladder, nerves and joints
PROPERTIES: Diuretic
Lithotriptic
Stimulant
Astringent
Nervine

Gravel root is highly regarded as a remedy for gravel and stones of the kidneys and bladder. It is also used to treat water retention and joint pains caused by uric acid deposits.

A strong decoction is used, with one ounce of the root boiled in a pint of water for one hour. The tea is taken a quarter cup at a time, as needed. The tincture may be used in doses of one teaspoon.

Gravel root is also commonly known as queen of the meadow and joe-pye root.

Hawthorn *Crataegus oxycantha*
Rosaceae

PART USED: Berries
SYSTEMS AFFECTED: Heart and circulation
PROPERTIES: Cardiac tonic
Diuretic
Astringent
antispasmodic
sedative

Hawthorn is well known for its effectiveness in treating both high and low blood pressure, rapid or arhythmic heartbeat, inflammation of the heart muscle and arteriosclerosis. Its regular use strengthens the heart muscle. Hawthorn is also very effective for relieving insomnia.

A decoction of the berries is useful for treating sore throats. The native Americans also used it to treat rheumatism. The tincture is also useful. Steep four ounces of the berries in a pint of brandy for two weeks and strain. The dose is fifteen drops, three times daily.

Horsetail *Equisetum arvense*
Equisetaceae

PART USED: Aboveground portion
SYSTEMS AFFECTED: Kidneys and blood
PROPERTIES: Diuretic
Astringent

Horsetail — cont'd
               Nutritive tonic
               Lithotriptic
               hemostatic
               vulnerary
               emmenagogue

Horsetail is a reliable diuretic and is used for all urinary disorders. A decoction of the shoots is taken in the quantity of one cup, two or three times a day, or two tablespoons every hour.

Horsetail helps coagulate blood and thus is useful to help stop bleeding. It also clears fevers, releases nervous tension and calms an overactive liver. Studies have shown that fractured bones will heal much faster when horsetail is taken. The early spring horsetail is the one that should be used.

Horsetail is rich in minerals, especially silica and selenium. Excessive use will irritate the kidneys and intestines; thus it is an herb best taken in frequent small doses and not for prolonged periods of time. Two or three weeks of treatment with horsetail should be followed by a week without its use, and then the treatment could be repeated if necessary.

The "scouring brush," as it is called, is ridged with silica and traditionally makes one of the finest scouring pads and abrasives, still preferred by fine cabinetmakers for polishing wood finishes.

Hyssop   *Hyssopus officinalis*
                                           Labiatae

PART USED: Leaves
SYSTEMS AFFECTED: Lungs, sinuses and blood
PROPERTIES: Expectorant
                  Diaphoretic
                  Stimulant
                  Vulnerary

Hyssop is used in the treatment of lung ailments, especially for chronic catarrh. It is a valuable expectorant and is used for coughs and congestion due to colds and flus. It is used for sweating to reduce fevers.

As a stimulant, hyssop helps promote circulation and improve sluggish digestion.

Externally, hyssop is applied to wounds to cure infection and help the tissue heal more rapidly.

Prepare hyssop as an infusion, using one ounce of herb per pint of water, or as a tincture, using four ounces of herb per pint of alcohol. The dose is one-half cup of tea or one teaspoon of the tincture, three times daily.

Irish moss   *Chondrus crispus*
Algae

PART USED: Whole plant
SYSTEMS AFFECTED: Lungs, kidneys and skin; general effects on
the whole body
PROPERTIES: Demulcent
Emollient
Nutritive tonic

Irish moss is very high in mucilage, making it an excellent demulcent for soothing inflamed tissues, and all lung and kidney complaints. It can be used externally to soften skin and prevent premature wrinkling.

Irish moss and other seaweeds are among the richest sources of minerals. Thus they are important nutritive tonics to be used in treating weakness and deficiencies.

Steep one-half ounce of Irish moss in cold water for fifteen minutes, then boil it in three pints of milk or water for ten to fifteen minutes, after which it is strained and seasoned with licorice, cinnamon and honey to taste. Drink one-half cup, three times daily, as a nutritive tonic and for all lung complaints.

Juniper   *Juniperis communis*
Coniferae

PART USED: Berries
SYSTEMS AFFECTED: Kidneys and stomach
PROPERTIES: Stimulant
Diuretic
Astringent
carminative
lithotriptic

Juniper berries are a stimulating diuretic, beneficial in the treatment of urine retention, gravel, pains in the lumbar region, bladder discharges and uric acid buildup. Four to six drops of the oil, taken with honey three or four times a day, has been a successful home remedy for these ailments. It is a useful carminative for indigestion and flatulence.

Large doses are irritating to the urinary tract. Juniper berries should not be used when there is inflammation of the kidneys.

Kava kava   *Known to damage liver*   *Piper methysticum*
Piperaceae

PART USED: Root
SYSTEMS AFFECTED: Nerves
PROPERTIES: Antispasmodic
Analgesic

Kava kava—cont'd
>Antiseptic
>Sedative
>Tonic
>Diuretic

Kava kava is a Polynesian herb that is excellent as a remedy for insomnia and nervousness. Taken at night, it invokes a deep restful sleep with clear, epic-length dreams. It is valuable to use when only a few hours sleep are possible.

Kava kava is a potent analgesic that may be taken internally or applied directly to a painful wound. It is also antiseptic and may be used as a douche for vaginitis. It is a valuable diuretic for treating urinary tract infections.

It is used in Polynesia as a beverage and as a daily tonic. However, regular use of large doses will cause an accumulation of toxic substances in the liver. It is safest to use by grinding the root and making an infusion. Combine four tablespoons crushed root with some flavoring herbs, such as peppermint and raspberry leaves, and steep ten minutes in a pint of boiled water.

Lady's slipper   *Cypredium pubescens*
                                                      Orchidaceae

PART USED: Root
SYSTEMS AFFECTED: Nerves
PROPERTIES: Nervine
>Antispasmodic
>Sedative

Lady's slipper is considered to be one of the purest and surest acting nervines that can be relied upon in the treatment of chorea, epilepsy, hysteria, headache, insomnia and general nervousness. It apparently has no narcotic properties.

Lady's slipper can be combined with ginger and a small amount of lobelia for the treatment of nervousness associated with fevers. It can be combined with dandelion or camomile for effective treatment of stomach or liver problems, including hepatitis.

For acute nervous affections, frequent small doses (two tablespoons) of the decoction, one ounce of the root per pint of water, should be taken every hour or as needed. Or the tincture can be made, and taken in doses of one teaspoon.

Lemon balm   *Melissa officinalis*
                                                  Labiatae

PART USED: Leaves
SYSTEMS AFFECTED: Nerves and circulation
PROPERTIES: Diaphoretic
            Antispasmodic
            Sedative
            Antipyretic

This is a great herb for all infants' and children's afflictions. It is the best tasting anti-fever tea and is useful for the first signs of colds, flus and fevers. Take copious amounts of the sweetened infusion, soak in a hot bath and retire to bed with several warm blankets in order to sweat it out.

This herb is widely used to cure melancholy and diseases that are the result of finding ourselves in places and life situations we are not ready to accept.

Prepare the infusion in a tightly covered vessel using an ounce of the herb per pint of water. Sweeten with honey to taste.

Lobelia   *Lobelia inflata*
                                                  Lobeliaceae

PART USED: Aboveground portion
SYSTEMS AFFECTED: Nerves, lungs, stomach, muscles and circu-
                 lation
PROPERTIES: Nervine
            Antispasmodic
            Emetic
            Expectorant

Lobelia is a very commonly used antispasmodic herb, applied both internally and externally to relax all spasms. In small doses (fifteen drops of the tincture, one gelatin capsule) lobelia is used for lung congestion and as an antispasmodic in herb formulas. In large doses (forty drops of the tincture, two gelatin capsules or more), it is used as a powerful emetic (see chapter on "Herbal Therapies").

Lobelia is applied externally in baths, fomentations, poultices and liniments for muscle spasms. A few drops of the tincture placed in the ear will relieve earaches. It is added to catnip in preparing an enema for fevers and infections. Lobelia can be smoked or taken internally to help break the habit of smoking tobacco.

Licorice *(See Chinese herb section)*

Malva   *Malva spp.*
                                                       Malvaceae

PART USED: Leaves, flowers and root
SYSTEMS AFFECTED: Blood, liver, lungs, urinary tract, stomach
                 and skin
PROPERTIES: Demulcent
            Emollient
            Diuretic
            astringent

Malva can be found growing almost everywhere. A tea of the leaves and flowers can be used to treat fevers, colds and all inflammatory conditions. The root is used to treat painful urination and the pains associated with the passage of either biliary or urinary stones. The leaves can be eaten in soups and stews, being a very good source of vitamins and minerals.

Externally, a poultice may be made of the leaves and flowers and applied to acute rashes, sprains and burns.

The properties of malva are similar to marshmallow, and the marshmallow is considered superior. However, malva is much more common and is a readily available first aid remedy.

The tea is made by steeping one ounce of the leaves and flowers in a pint of boiled water, or making a decoction of the root using similar quantities. The tincture is also used, in doses of two teaspoons as needed.

Mandrake   *Podophyllum peltatum*
                                                Berberidaceae

PART USED: Root
SYSTEMS AFFECTED: Liver, gallbladder, intestines and skin
PROPERTIES: Laxative
            Hepatic tonic
            Alterative
            Emetic
            Cholagogue
            Stimulant

Mandrake is a very powerful glandular stimulant that should be taken in small doses and with great respect for its potency. It is excellent for the treatment of chronic liver diseases, skin eruptions, bile imbalances and obstructions in digestion and elimination. It is best taken in small doses in combination with such supporting herbs as Oregon grape root, ginger or licorice. Use one capsule or fifteen drops of the tincture.

Externally, the concentrated tincture (obtained by gently cooking down the tincture) is directly applied to warts to help rapidly remove them. A prescription drug, podophyllin, is this resinous black extract, and is commonly prescribed for venereal warts. Care should be taken to apply this only to the wart and to avoid contact with the surrounding skin. Large doses, even applied externally, are toxic.

Marshmallow   *Althea officinalis*
                                                        Malvaceae

PART USED: Root
SYSTEMS AFFECTED: Intestines, kidneys and bladder; general
                effects on the whole body
PROPERTIES: Demulcent
            Emollient
            Alterative
            diuretic
            vulnerary
            nutritional tonic
            lithotriptic

Marshmallow is the best source of easily-digested vegetable mucilage. This mucilage will aid the body's mucus in lubricating the joints to protect them against irritation and dryness and in regulating the heat of the body. Our digestive fluids are also associated with a mucousy quality that is assisted by the mucilage of marshmallow. Marshmallow is thus a powerful antiinflammatory and an anti-irritant for the joints and the gastrointestinal tract. It is also of value for all lung ailments.

Used in combination with other diuretic herbs, such as parsley root, in the form of a tea, marshmallow root will relieve the attack of kidney stone and gravel and aid in their smooth expulsion. It can be used with other laxative herbs for chronic constipation that is associated with dryness or lack of roughage. Marshmallow is also protective and healing in the irritations associated with diarrhea and dysentery.

Applied externally as a poultice on a daily basis, marshmallow root with a pinch of cayenne can be relied upon to treat blood poisoning, gangrene, septic wounds, burns and bruises.

Marshmallow is high in minerals, especially easily assimilable calcium. It is taken as an ingredient in herb teas, or in gelatin capsules or pills, usually as 10% of the formula.

Motherwort   *Leonurus cardiaca*
                                                 Labiatae

PART USED: Aboveground portion
SYSTEMS AFFECTED: Nerves, heart and uterus
PROPERTIES: Nervine
            Cardiac tonic
            Emmenagogue
            Antispasmodic
            diaphoretic
            laxative

Motherwort is a very useful herb to treat suppressed menstruation
and other female disorders. A good combination of herbs for this
purpose is motherwort with cramp bark and calendula in equal parts.

Motherwort is a good tonic for the heart and may be combined with
hawthorn berries for a very effective heart tonic and antispasmodic.
This can be used to prevent heart attack and to treat palpitations
and neuralgia.

It is excellent for treating nervous conditions such as hysteria, convulsions and insomnia. Motherwort is used by making an infusion
with one ounce of the herb per pint of water. The tincture may also
be used, in doses of one-half teaspoon, three times daily.

Mugwort   *Artemisia vulgaris*
                                                 Compositae

PART USED: Leaves
SYSTEMS AFFECTED: Nerves, circulation, stomach and uterus
PROPERTIES: Nervine
            Emmenagogue
            Diuretic
            Diaphoretic
            Stomach tonic

Mugwort is an excellent nervine for uncontrollable shaking, nervousness and insomnia. It may be taken as tea, using an ounce of the
herb to a pint of water, steeped twenty minutes. The dose is one tablespoon three times daily. Mugwort can also be smoked, filling the lungs
three to six times.

The tea is also useful for treating stomach disorders, and for this
purpose it is diluted three times to overcome the strong taste. The
native Americans used the tea for colds and flus, bronchitis and
fevers. It may be taken hot for sweating therapy. Mugwort will bring
on the menstrual period and is commonly used with other herbs,
such as cramp bark, for the treatment of menstrual cramps and other
female problems.

Wormwood (*Artemisia absinthium*) has many similar properties, being used as a nervine and stomach tonic. It is used in the same way, as a tea, but taken in half-cup doses.

Mullein   *Verbascum thapsus*
                                                     Scrophulariaceae

PART USED: Leaves and flowers
SYSTEMS AFFECTED: Lungs, glands and lymph
PROPERTIES: Expectorant
           Astringent
           Diuretic
           Vulnerary
           demulcent
           antispasmodic

Mullein may be smoked for the treatment of congestion of the lungs and for coughs. A tea (infusion) is made, combining mullein with yerba santa, wild cherry bark, licorice and comfrey root, for these conditions.

Mullein leaves are used to treat lymphatic congestion that results in earaches, toothaches and hemorrhoids. It is also useful in the treatment of diarrhea.

One of the most common uses of mullein flowers is as a nervine and antispasmodic. The oil is considered one of the best for all ear complaints, applied a few drops in the ear overnight.

Myrrh   *Commiphora myrrha*
                                                   Burseraceae

PART USED: Resin
SYSTEMS AFFECTED: Stomach and lungs; general effects on the
                       whole body
PROPERTIES: Antiseptic
           Astringent
           Stimulant
           expectorant
           carminative
           emmenagogue

Myrrh gum is one of the most effective of the botanical antiseptics. It is often combined with an equal amount of goldenseal to make a healing antiseptic salve, useful in treating hemorrhoids, bed sores and wounds. A tincture of myrrh gum makes an excellent mouthwash good for spongy gums, pyrrohea, sore throat and other ailments requiring an astringent.

Internally, myrrh gum is used to treat indigestion and gas, and it is an excellent treatment for chronic catarrh and bronchial congestion. It is valuable for treating ulcers.

Other gums and resinous materials from conifers such as pine and fir have similar properties. An elderly healer in northern California was very highly regarded for her ability to cure arthritis, skin diseases and indigestion using resins from the local trees.

Myrrh and other gums should be used in small amounts internally as they contain potent volatile oils that are toxic in large amounts. Small doses of the gums will help remove toxins from the stomach and intestines. Use the tincture, thirty drops each time, or the powder in capsules or pills, one or two each time, as needed.

Nettles   *Urtica urens*
                                                                 Urticaceae

PART USED: Leaves
SYSTEMS AFFECTED: Lungs, kidneys, bladder and blood
PROPERTIES: Expectorant
            Alterative
            Hemostatic
            antiseptic

Nettles is considered a specific for asthma when taken over a prolonged period. I often combine it with equal parts of comfrey, mullein and a pinch of lobelia. A tea made from this simple formula, using an ounce of herbs steeped in a pint of boiled water, is taken three to four times a day. Its effects are to provide an expectorant, an antispasmodic and an aid to the assimilation of important minerals. Nettles is very rich in iron, silicon and potassium.

Nettles tea is a safe remedy for bleeding and anemia, and it is a useful blood purifier. It may be applied externally, by sprinkling some nettle powder directly on the affected area, to help stop bleeding.

The fresh young leaves, carefully picked with gloves, make a highly nutritious vegetable when steamed. The expressed juice is made by bruising the leaves and subjecting them to low heat for thirty minutes, then wringing them out in a cloth. Take one tablespoon of this juice in one-half cup water every hour to stop bleeding. This juice is also applied to the scalp for stimulating hair growth. The antidote to poisoning from nettle sting is fresh yellow dock or plantain leaves bruised and rubbed over the affected area.

Oregon grape root *Berberis aquifolium*
Berberidaceae

PART USED: Rhizome and root
SYSTEMS AFFECTED: Liver, stomach, intestines, blood and skin
PROPERTIES: Biliary tonic
Alterative
Laxative
antiseptic

Oregon grape root stimulates the production of bile and thus aids in digestion and purifying the blood. A teaspoon of the tincture, taken three to four times daily, is taken for the treatment of all skin diseases due to toxins in the blood, including psoriasis, eczema, herpes and acne. It is also useful in treating rheumatoid arthritis and hepatitis.

Oregon grape root is almost identical to barberry (*Berberis vulgaris*) in its action, but has a stronger effect on the liver and has a stimulating action on the thyroid. It is a tonic for all the glands and it aids in the assimilation of nutrients.

Oregon grape root has been used in the treatment of bronchial congestion. It has mild antiseptic effects and is thus useful in douches for vaginitis.

Parsley *Petroselinum* spp.
Umbelliferae

PART USED: Leaves and root
SYSTEMS AFFECTED: Kidneys, bladder, stomach, liver and
gallbladder
PROPERTIES: Diuretic
Tonic
Nervine
carminative
expectorant

Parsley leaves have repeatedly proved useful for bladder infections, especially if taken in combination with equal parts of echinacea and marshmallow root. However, parsley is a warming herb and should generally be avoided when there are other acute infections and inflammations present, especially of the kidneys.

Parsley root and leaves are both good for the removal of all stones, including gallstones, if they are not too large. The root is particularly useful for treating chronic diseases and ailments of the liver and

gallbladder. It can be used with a small amount of licorice or marshmallow root for the treatment of jaundice, asthma, water retention
and coughs.

The leaf is best taken fresh, as a salad vegetable. The root is prepared as a decoction, usually in combination with other roots, such as
dandelion, chicory and burdock, making a total of one ounce of roots
per pint of water simmered for about one hour. Take one-half cup of
the tea, three times daily.

Pennyroyal   *Mentha pulegium*
                                                  Labiatae

PART USED: Aboveground portion
SYSTEMS AFFECTED: Circulation, uterus and lungs
PROPERTIES: Diaphoretic
            Stimulant
            Emmenagogue
            carminative

Pennyroyal is a very good herb to use for all fevers and lung infections. It drives out the heat and inflammation through the pores of the
skin and helps the circulation. Pennyroyal is good for the treatment
of nervous headaches.

A tea has been used to induce abortions, but serious consequences
follow from using the essential oil internally for this purpose. It is
useful in regulation of the menstrual flow and for relieving cramps.
It should not be used by those who have a tendency toward excessive
menstruation.

Pennyroyal is a very strong smelling mint and it is used externally
to repel insects such as fleas, mosquitos and flies.

The American species, *Hedeoma pulegioides,* and the European
species, *Mentha pulegium,* share very similar properties. Prepare an
infusion using one ounce of pennyroyal per pint of water. Use one-
half cup of the tea as needed, or a cup of the tea to induce sweating.

Plantain   *Plantago* spp.
                                                  Plantaginaceae

PART USED: Leaves and seeds
SYSTEMS AFFECTED: General effect on all systems
PROPERTIES: Vulnerary
            Astringent
            Diuretic
            emollient
            antiseptic
            expectorant

The cooling, soothing properties of plantain account for its effectiveness in a wide range of ailments, including: diarrhea, hemorrhoids, infections and inflammations, ulcers, bronchitis and excessive menstrual discharge. Make an infusion using an ounce of the herb in a pint of water. It will also neutralize stomach acids and normalize all stomach secretions. The seeds (known as psyllium seeds) are a useful bulk laxative, one-half ounce taken with a cup of hot water.

Essentially all the plantains have similar properties, but the wider the leaf the more pronounced the diuretic effect. It is useful in the treatment of water retention and kidney and bladder infections.

Plantain is commonly known to relieve the pain and neutralize the toxins of insect and snake bites. Take a fresh leaf or two, chew it slightly and then apply directly to the bite. It is used in a variety of salves and ointments, alone or in combination with other herbs such as chickweed, comfrey, elder flowers, mugwort and angelica. It is one of the best remedies for cuts, skin infections and chronic skin problems.

Poke *Phytolacca americana*
Phytolaccaceae

PART USED: Root
SYSTEMS AFFECTED: Blood, lymph and lungs
PROPERTIES: Alterative
           Anticatarrhal
           Laxative
           Emetic

Poke root is commonly used in small doses as a blood purifier in combination with others possessing this property, such as red clover, echinacea and yellow dock. It stimulates elimination, being a laxative in large doses and an emetic in very large doses. It reduces inflammation and is used for rheumatism, tonsillitis, laryngitis and mumps.

Poke is also used for chronic catarrh and respiratory tract diseases. It aids in clearing the lymph.

Externally, poke is applied as a salve to treat scabies, acne and fungal infections, and as a poultice for abscesses.

Poke root contains toxic mitogenic substances and therefore must be used in small quantities, not to exceed about one gram per day. It is usually taken in capsules or as a tincture. The fresh root is much more potent than the dried root and, when available, is included in small amounts in a tea with other herbs such as red clover.

Prickly Ash   *Xanthoxylum americanum*
                                             Rutaceae
PART USED: Bark
SYSTEMS AFFECTED: Blood, circulation and stomach
PROPERTIES: Stimulant
              Alterative
              Antispasmodic
              Astringent
              emmenagogue
              rubefacient

Prickly ash bark is a stimulant that greatly increases the circulation throughout the body. It is thus used in most cases of impaired circulation, including cold extremities and joints, rheumatism and arthritis, lethargy and wounds that are slow to heal. In addition, it is a blood purifier, useful in treating skin diseases and accumulations in the joints.

Prickly ash is very warming to the stomach and is thus useful for weak digestion, as well as colic and cramps.

A decoction is made by boiling an ounce of the bark in three pints of water, until the liquid is reduced to about one pint. This is taken in frequent doses, totaling two cups per day. It is an excellent herb to add as the stimulant in a formula for acute ailments, superior to cayenne, black pepper or ginger for this purpose.

Externally, prickly ash is applied as a poultice to help dry up and heal wounds. The bark powder can be chewed for relief of toothaches.

As a stimulant astringent, prickly ash bark is very similar to bayberry bark.

Prince's pine (Pipsissewa)   *Chimaphila umbellata*
                                             Ericacea
PART USED: Leaves
SYSTEMS AFFECTED: Genitourinary, liver, skin and circulation
PROPERTIES: Diuretic
              Astringent
              laxative

Prince's pine is useful in the treatment of all urinary and genital infections, its action being similar to, and somewhat milder than, uva ursi. It is excellent for the treatment of skin diseases resulting from faulty elimination through the urinary tract. As such it is one of the best remedies for arthritis and rheumatism. I have seen Karok Indian women in their late eighties drinking a quart or two of prince's pine tea a day for stiffness and genitourinary problems.

Prince's pine is a mild laxative and thus is an excellent remedy for most diseases, as it will tend to tonify and promote normal elimina-

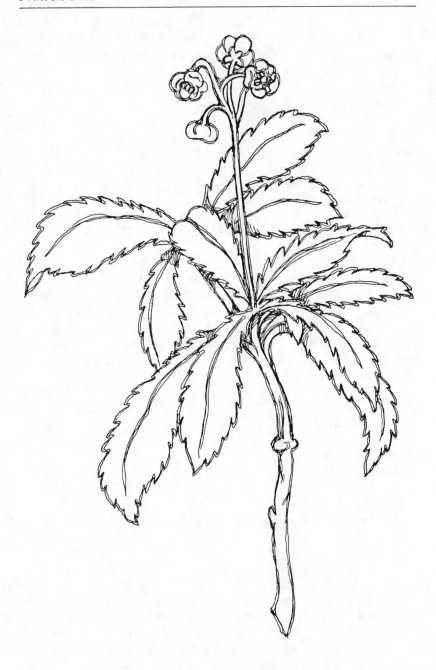

PRINCE'S PINE (*Chimaphila umbellata*)

Useful in the treatment of all urinary and genital infections.

tion. For most liver, kidney, joint and skin problems, a combination of Oregon grape root and prince's pine taken frequently throughout the day will prove very helpful.

It is taken either as an infusion, an extract in wine or a tincture and it may be used freely, as needed.

Raspberry   *Rubus idaeus*
                                                   Rosaceae

PART USED: Leaves
SYSTEMS AFFECTED: Stomach, liver, blood, genitourinary tract
               and muscles
PROPERTIES: Antispasmodic
            Astringent
            stimulant

Raspberry leaf tea is one of the most renowned herbal teas for pregnancy, relieving nausea, preventing hemorrhage, reducing pain and easing childbirth. It is also used freely to reduce menstrual cramps. It is combined with other herbs, such as uva ursi and squaw-vine, for the treatment of vaginal discharge and other female disorders.

Raspberry is also a reliable treatment for acute stomach problems, fevers, colds and flus.

The tea is made by steeping an ounce of the herb in a pint of boiled water for twenty minutes. The tincture may also be used in doses of two tablespoons.

Rhubarb   *Rheum palmatum*
                                                   Polygonaceae

PART USED: Root
SYSTEMS AFFECTED: Stomach and intestines
PROPERTIES: Astringent
            Alterative
            Stomach tonic
            sialagogue

Rhubarb is one of the best herbs for treating diarrhea and dysentery caused by an irritating body in the intestines. Turkey rhubarb is the most valuable species. It acts as a laxative, clearing the cause of intestinal irritation and checking diarrhea with its astringent action. In small doses, it acts to aid digestion and is an effective tonic for the stomach and other digestive organs. When chewed, it acts to stimulate the flow of saliva.

Rhubarb is also considered a very Yin tonic in Chinese medicine, useful in treating most Yang conditions, especially toxic blood conditions from excessive intake of meat and other Yang foods.

Rhubarb may be taken as a powder in gelatin capsules, one to three capsules each time, depending on the use (three capsules for a laxative effect). The tincture is taken in teaspoon quantities, up to a tablespoon for the treatment of amoebic dysentery.

Rue *Ruta graveolens*
Rutaceae

PART USED: Aboveground portion
SYSTEMS AFFECTED: Nerves, tendons, circulation and uterus
PROPERTIES: Antispasmodic
Emmenagogue
Stimulant
Rubefacient

Rue is a valuable antispasmodic herb useful in the treatment of hypertension, nervous complaints, neuralgia, trauma and cramps. It seems to exert a strong influence on the tendons and is widely prescribed by homeopaths as a first aid medicine for strained tendons and muscles.

The Chinese use a tincture of rue for sedation, for decreasing swelling, for rheumatism, for increasing local circulation and for improving metabolism.

Rue tincture can be taken in small doses of one-half to one teaspoon at a time, but should be used in moderation. If there are any adverse symptoms of overdose, a small amount of goldenseal root will act as an antidote. Because rue has emmenagogue properties, it should be avoided by all pregnant women. Rue is used externally as a rubefacient to promote local circulation.

Sarsaparilla *Smilax ornata*
Liliaceae

PART USED: Root
SYSTEMS AFFECTED: Blood, skin, circulation and intestines
PROPERTIES: Alterative
Carminative
Diaphoretic

Sarsaparilla root is useful in the treatment of gout, rheumatism, colds, fevers and catarrhal problems, as well as other ailments requiring a good blood purifier. It is used externally for the treatment of skin problems, including skin parasites.

The hot decoction, made with an ounce of root in a pint of water, will promote profuse sweating and will act as a powerful agent to expel gas from the stomach and intestines.

Sarsaparilla contains hormone-like substances and thus is valuable in glandular balance formulas. It is frequently combined with sassafras and a little yellow dock as a spring tonic and blood purifier.

Sassafras   *Sassafras officinale*
                                                 Lauraceae

PART USED: Root bark
SYSTEMS AFFECTED: Liver, blood and skin
PROPERTIES: Alterative
            Diuretic
            Diaphoretic
            Stimulant
            Hepatic tonic
            Astringent

Sassafras is one of the oldest and most highly respected remedies of North America. It is considered to be a spring tonic, and an excellent blood purifier. Sassafras stimulates the action of the liver to clear toxins from the system. It is often combined with other alteratives, such as sarsaparilla, licorice, burdock and echinacea, for chronic blood disorders.

Its action on the blood explains its usefulness as a treatment for all skin disorders, especially eruptions such as acne. Sassafras is also a powerful diuretic.

Sassafras tea is made by boiling the root bark in a covered pot for twenty minutes, using one-half ounce of the herb per pint of water. It is taken in quantities of one-half cup, three times daily. Larger quantities may cause overstimulation of the liver and a toxic reaction. Sassafras is high in tannins and can be taken with milk to reduce the astringent effects. The oil is used externally for rheumatic pains but should not be used internally.

Senna   *Cassia acutifolia*
                                                 Leguminosae

PART USED: Leaves and pods
SYSTEMS AFFECTED: Intestines
PROPERTIES: Laxative

Senna is one of the most reliable laxatives. It increases the intestinal peristaltic movements. Senna must be taken with carminative herbs such as ginger, cardamon, coriander or fennel to prevent griping (bowel cramps). Use an ounce of senna per pint of water, with about 10% ginger or other carminative. Steep for fifteen minutes in a covered vessel, and drink cool. Do not make up more than is to be used—about one-half to one cup at a time, as needed. Alternatively, use two gelatin capsules of the powder or one teaspoon of the tincture. The pods are milder than the leaves and less likely to cause griping.

Skullcap *Scutellaria* spp.
Labiatae

PART USED: Aboveground portion
SYSTEMS AFFECTED: Nerves and stomach
PROPERTIES: Nervine
        Antipyretic
        Antispasmodic

Skullcap is a very safe and reliable nerve sedative. It is good for drug and alcoholic withdrawal symptoms, hysteria, epilepsy, neuralgia, convulsions, hypertension, insomnia and restlessness. Skullcap is food for the nerves, supporting and strengthening them as it gives immediate relief of all chronic and acute diseases stemming from nervous affections and debility. Skullcap is combined with great advantage with other tonic nervine and antispasmodic herbs, such as hops, passion flower, lady's slipper and wood betony.

Skullcap is high in calcium, potassium and magnesium, accounting for many of its remarkable effects in quieting the entire nervous system. It may be used freely, as it is essentially nontoxic. Use an ounce of the herb, steeped in a pint of boiled water for ten minutes.

Slippery Elm *Ulmus fulva*
Ulmaceae

PART USED: Inner bark
SYSTEMS AFFECTED: General effects on the whole body
PROPERTIES: Demulcent
        Emollient
        Nutritive tonic
        astringent

Powdered slippery elm can be made into a gruel by gradually adding a small amount of water and mixing until the proper consistency is obtained. This can be sweetened with a little honey, and a dash of cinnamon, cloves and other spices can be added for their flavor and therapeutic value. It is an excellent food whenever there is difficulty holding and digesting food. It will heal stomach and intestinal ulcers very quickly, and normalizes bowel function to relieve constipation and diarrhea. Slippery elm will also soothe inflamed lungs and is very beneficial in the treatment of coughs and bronchitis, especially when combined with licorice.

The mucilage of slippery elm works as an excellent binder. A small amount added to other herbs with a little water can be rolled into small pills; lozenges for coughs and sore throats can be made by adding a little maple syrup to the slippery elm; suppositories and boluses are made using slippery elm as a binder.

Externally, the moistened slippery elm can be applied to sores, wounds, gangrene, burns, tumors and infected areas. It is an excellent cleanser and can be used in a douche or enema.

Spearmint   *Mentha viridis*
                                                       Labiatae

PART USED: Leaves
SYSTEMS AFFECTED: Stomach, intestines, muscles and circulation
PROPERTIES: Diaphoretic
            Carminative
            Stimulant
            Antispasmodic
            Diaphoretic

Spearmint is useful for all minor ailments, including colds, flus, fevers, indigestion, gas, cramps and spasms. Peppermint *(Mentha piperita)* has the same herbal properties except that it is more stimulating. Both are commonly used as flavoring agents in herbal teas. The menthol found in these plants is a stimulating diaphoretic. A mixture of elder flowers and mints makes an excellent tea for sweating therapy.

For a beverage tea, use the mints alone or in combination with mild herbs, using one-half ounce of herb per pint of water. For a medicinal tea, double the quantity of herbs.

Squawvine   *Mitchella repens*
                                                       Rubiaceae

PART USED: Leaves and berries
SYSTEMS AFFECTED: Uterus, bladder and colon
PROPERTIES: Uterine tonic
            Astringent
            Diuretic

Squawvine is useful for the treatment of water retention, diarrhea, gravel and leukorrhea. It is considered very helpful for the uterus, especially to facilitate childbirth. Externally it is used as a wash for sore eyes.

Combined with wild yam, raspberry leaves and a small portion of lobelia, squawvine is used to prevent miscarriages. The same formula may prove beneficial in the treatment of bladder infections and vaginal discharges.

Squawvine is similar in action to prince's pine. One-half cup of the tea is taken three times a day, made as the decoction, using an ounce of herb in a pint of water. The tincture is taken one tablespoon each dose.

Stoneroot *Collinsonia canadensis*
Labiatae

PART USED: Root
SYSTEMS AFFECTED: Veins, liver and colon
PROPERTIES: Astringent
　　　　　　 Diuretic
　　　　　　 Hepatic tonic

Stoneroot is primarily used in the treatment of hemorrhoids. Its astringency focuses on restoring the tone of flaccid veins and it is thus useful for both hemorrhoids and varicose veins. It can be taken internally as a tincture, one teaspoon three times daily, or in gelatin capsules, two capsules three times daily. Externally, it is applied directly to hemorrhoids in a salve with equal parts goldenseal and a small amount of thuja oil or tea tree oil.

Stoneroot is also used for treating both diarrhea and constipation. It can be used with gravel root in the removal of bladder stones. Small amounts are useful for treating hoarse voice. If used in large doses it may cause nausea.

Uva ursi (Bearberry) *Arctostaphylos uva ursi*
Ericacea

PART USED: Leaves
SYSTEMS AFFECTED: Kidneys and urinary tract
PROPERTIES: Astringent
　　　　　　 Diuretic
　　　　　　 Alterative

Uva ursi is a specific for the treatment of bladder and kidney infections, and when combined with marshmallow root, is useful for eliminating stones from those organs. Tincture of uva ursi was routinely prescribed in many European hospitals as a postpartum medicine to reduce hemorrhaging and help restore the womb to normal size.

The common manzanita *(Arctostaphylos* spp.*)* can be used for the same purposes, though uva ursi is considered to be better because of its milder nature. Prepare the infusion, with one ounce of herb per pint of water, or the tincture, using four ounces of herb per pint of alcohol. Uva ursi is commonly combined with buchu leaves.

Valerian *Valeriana officinalis*
Valerianaceae

PART USED: Root
SYSTEMS AFFECTED: Nerves
PROPERTIES: Nervine
　　　　　　 Antispasmodic

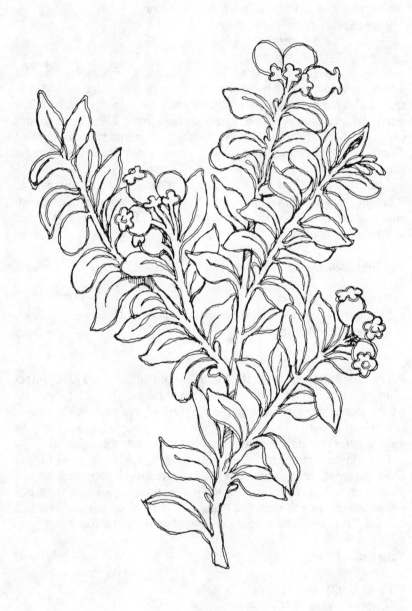

UVA URSI (*Arctostaphylos uva ursi*)

A specific for the treatment of bladder and kidney infections.

Valerian is considered to be very sedating and calming for all emotional disturbances and pain. A few individuals may find that valerian can have a stimulating effect. This is because the essential oil of valerian was not transformed by the body's own enzymes into valerianic acid, the calming principle. It will have a stimulating effect until that enzymatic process occurs.

Valerian can be combined with many other herbs to add a tonic, antispasmodic nervine property and thus it is widely used in many nervine formulas. One of the classic bedtime teas for insomnia is one-half teaspoon valerian root and one-half teaspoon hops steeped in a cup of hot water.

Valerian should not be boiled, as this will dissipate the essential oils that contain the primary therapeutic ingredients.

Hops *(Humulus lupulus)* has very similar properties and may be substituted. Used in a pillow, it is a classic treatment for insomnia.

Vervain   *Verbena officinalis*
Verbenaceae

PART USED: Flowers and leaves
SYSTEMS AFFECTED: Circulation, lungs and intestines
PROPERTIES: Antipyretic
Diaphoretic
Expectorant
Astringent
Antispasmodic

Vervain is an excellent herb to use for fevers, especially in combination with boneset. It is taken as a hot tea every hour and will induce sweating. It is also useful for colds, flus and coughs.

It is used in treating most lung ailments, and will greatly aid in expelling mucus. It is also good for nervous conditions and headaches.

Vervain is a popular remedy for griping (intestinal cramps).

White oak   *Quercus alba*
Fagaceae

PART USED: Bark
SYSTEMS AFFECTED: Skin; general effects on the whole body
PROPERTIES: Astringent

White oak bark is one of the most widely used astringents. It can be used for internal treatments such as ulcers, spleen problems and diarrhea. Externally it is applied to wounds, poison oak and insect and snake bites. It may be used in a douche for vaginal infections. Applied to the gums, it will tighten them and prevent the loss of teeth. Simmer an ounce of the bark in a pint of water for an hour.

Wild yam   *Dioscorea villosa*
                                                     Dioscoreaceae

PART USED: Rhizome and root
SYSTEMS AFFECTED: Muscles, joints, uterus, liver and gallbladder
PROPERTIES: Antispasmodic
            Cholagogue
            diaphoretic

Wild yam contains substances related to human steroid hormones
and is used as a source for steroids used in birth control pills and
cortisone treatments. These hormone substances make wild yam a
useful ingredient in glandular balance formulas and for treating
nausea for pregnant women.

Wild yam is a valuable antispasmodic for treating griping (bowel
spasms), hiccough, menstrual cramps and muscle pain. It is used in
the treatment of arthritis and inflammations of the joints.

As a stimulant to the bile, it is useful in the treatment of bilious
colic. It is very useful in the correction of intestinal gas.

Wild yam is used in small quantities, as an ingredient in herb tea
formulas or taken in capsules, two each time, three times daily.

Witch hazel   *Haemamelis virginiana*
                                                     Hamamelidaceae

PART USED: Leaves and bark
SYSTEMS AFFECTED: Skin, stomach and intestines; general effects
                 on the whole body
PROPERTIES: Astringent
            Tonic
            Hemostatic
            sedative

Witch hazel is mostly used externally as an alcohol extract applied
to insect bites, varicose veins, burns, hemmorhoids and to wounds
to stop bleeding. It may be used internally to help stop bleeding from
the lungs, uterus and other internal organs and in the treatment of
diarrhea. The extract, made by soaking an ounce of the leaves and
stems in a one pint mixture of equal parts of gin and water to which is
added a drop or two of peppermint oil, is used as a refreshing mouthwash. The mouthwash is helpful for sore throats and inflamed gums.

Wood betony   *Betonica officinalis*
                                                     Labiatae

PART USED: Aboveground portion
SYSTEMS AFFECTED: Nerves and liver
PROPERTIES: Nervine
            Alterative

Parasiticide

Analgesic

Betony is of great value for treating headaches, hysteria and other nervous afflictions. In addition, it is useful in treating diarrhea. A snuff made from the powders of equal parts of wood betony and marjoram, with a pinch of eyebright, is said to cure the most subborn headaches.

A strong decoction of wood betony will kill worms, open obstructions of the liver and gallbladder and relieve back pains and stitches in the side.

Betony is most frequently used in combination with other nervines to calm the nerves. It also benefits the function of the liver.

Wood betony is commonly used as a substitute for black tea. It shares a similar flavor, but lacks the caffeine and harmful acids. For this purpose, use one-half ounce of wood betony and steep in a pint of boiled water for ten minutes.

Yarrow
Achillea millefolium
Compositae

PART USED: Aboveground portion

SYSTEMS AFFECTED: General effects on the whole body

PROPERTIES: Diaphoretic

Astringent

Hemostatic

stimulant

Yarrow is a good herb for the early stages of flu and cold. It is also given to children for measles and other eruptive diseases, as a strong infusion.

Yarrow is rich in essential oils that are antiseptic and tannins, which are astringent. It can be applied directly to wounds to stop bleeding and is used in making a bolus or salve for bleeding piles. It relieves cramps and helps to stop excess menstrual bleeding when taken as a warm infusion. Use an ounce of the herb steeped in a pint of boiled water for twenty minutes.

Yellow dock
Rumex crispus
Polygonaceae

PART USED: Root

SYSTEMS AFFECTED: Blood, skin, stomach, spleen, liver and gallbladder

PROPERTIES: Astringent

Alterative

Laxative

Yellowdock — cont'd
                    Cholagogue
                    Nutritive tonic

Yellow dock is an astringent blood purifier useful in treating diseases of the blood and chronic skin ailments. It stimulates digestion, improving the function of the stomach and liver, and also stimulates elimination, improving flow of bile and acting as a laxative.

It is a nutritive tonic, high in iron and useful in treating anemia. It also nourishes the spleen and liver, thus being effective for the treatment of jaundice, lymphatic problems and skin eruptions.

Externally, it is applied as an astringent to bleeding piles, wounds and swellings.

It may be added in small amounts to herb tea formulas or taken in gelatin capsules, one or two capsules each time.

Yerba santa   *Eriodictyon californicum*
                                                   Hydrophyllaceae

PART USED: Leaves
SYSTEMS AFFECTED: Lungs and stomach
PROPERTIES: Expectorant
            Astringent
            Stimulant

Yerba santa is used for all forms of bronchial congestion, as it stimulates the salivary and other digestive secretions, thus correcting the congestion where it is usually caused — in the stomach. It is an excellent remedy for both acute and chronic chest conditions, including asthma. Combine with equal parts of mullein, nettles, comfrey root and a small amount of licorice in a tea.

Yerba santa is a good treatment for diarrhea and dysentery as well as common diseases such as colds and flus. It can be used in herbal smoking mixtures, with coltsfoot and mullein, for bronchial spasms.

Chinese Herbs

China is perhaps unique in the world in its long commitment to preventive medicine through the use of herbal tonics. The tonic herbs have several uses, including direct treatment of acute ailments, building strength in the recovery process, balancing the body's energy and preventing disease from occurring. These herbs are combined to make tonic soups providing nourishment and gentle stimulation to the organs. The Chinese herbs are becoming more readily available in the West, and many of the ones described here can be purchased in herb stores around the United States.

To make the herbal soup, combine six to seven grams (about one-quarter ounce) of each of the desired herbs in a large nonmetallic pot. Use a quart of water per ounce of herbs and simmer for an hour. Drink one cup of the tea, once per day, reheating the soup each day until it is all used. Always include some licorice in the formula.

Aconite (Fu tzu)   *Aconite fischeri*
                                               Ranunculaciae

PARTS USED: The prepared root
SYSTEMS AFFECTED: Nervous system, circulation, spleen, urinary system, heart and small intestine
PROPERTIES: Antispasmodic
                  Analgesic
                  Stimulant
                  Diuretic
                  Diaphoretic
                  Tonic

Aconite is considered the most Yang of all Oriental herbs. Because of its powerful Yang properties, it should be avoided, or used with caution, by those with a Yang condition. It can be toxic if used to excess. Much of the toxic properties of aconite have been neutralized by the Chinese in their processing and preparing the herb for medicine. It is used for Yin, weak people, and will stimulate sexual potency and relieve flatulence, excess moisture, coldness, numbness, pain, arthritis, sciatica and other severely painful conditions.

This herb is always used in combination with other herbs such as ginseng or licorice, or to balance Yin, eliminative herbs. In any case, it is never used in a dosage of more than two grams or so and is not prescribed for individuals who are hypertensives (have high blood pressure).

Externally, aconite is made into a liniment applied locally for the relief of neuralgia and rheumatism.

Astragalus   *Astragalus hoantchy*
                                               Leguminosae

PART USED: Root
SYSTEMS AFFECTED: Spleen, kidneys, lungs and blood
PROPERTIES: Stimulant
                  Diuretic
                  Tonic

Astragalus is used to increase the energy and build resistance to weakness and disease. It has warming properties and is tonic to the spleen, kidneys, lungs and blood.

Astragalus is combined with other herbs to promote their effects. It is a valuable diuretic.

Astragalus balances the energy of all the internal organs. It helps neutralize fevers and improves digestion.

It is one of the most valuable tonics, being used especially for those under thirty-five years of age. It is a specific for all wasting and exhausting diseases because it strengthens the body's resistance.

Chrysanthemum (Chinese)   *Chrysanthemum sinense*
                                                Compositae

PART USED: Flowers
SYSTEMS AFFECTED: Blood, nerves, digestion and liver
PROPERTIES: Alterative
            Antipyretic
            Carminative

Chrysanthemum flowers are valuable to counteract inflammation and pneumonia and in the treatment of fevers, headaches and dizziness. It helps purify the blood, calm the liver and brighten the eyes. Chrysanthemum is used to reduce inflammation, abscesses and boils. It is a cooling herb very popular in China for treating many Yang ailments.

Chrysanthemum is a carminative and is made into a healthful summer beverage in China.

Dong quai   *Angelica sinensis*
                                                Umbelliferae

PART USED: Root
SYSTEMS AFFECTED: Uterus, blood and muscles
PROPERTIES: Uterine tonic
            Antispasmodic
            Alterative

Dong quai is used for the treatment of almost every female gynecological ailment. It is particularly useful for the treatment of menstrual cramps, irregularity, delayed flow and weakness during the menstrual period. It is also used to relieve the symptoms of menopause.

Dong quai is a useful antispasmodic for treating insomnia, hypertension and cramps. It is nourishing to the blood and useful in treating anemia. Dong quai is a valuable blood purifier. It is warming to the circulation and is used to moisten the intestines to treat constipation.

Dong quai, also known as tang kwei, should not be used during pregnancy, or with excessive menstrual flow.

The Western herb angelica, *Angelica archangelica*, can be substituted in some cases. However, its action is harsher and it is a stimulant that reduces cramping through its warming quality, while dong quai accomplishes this through its antispasmodic components. Both are useful blood purifiers.

Don sen (Tang shen)   *Campanumaea pilosula*
                                           Campanulaceae
PART USED: Root
SYSTEMS AFFECTED: Spleen, pancreas, heart and stomach
PROPERTIES: Spleen tonic
          Stomach tonic

Don sen is used to strengthen the vital energy (*chi*) and is considered to be close in its properties to ginseng. It has the advantage of being cheaper, as well as useful at any time of year in both cold and warm climates, and it can be taken on a daily basis by both men and women. Its action is milder and safer than ginseng and it can be used for a longer treatment. It is recommended in combination with astragalus for increasing energy and building resistance to disease.

Don sen strengthens the functions of the spleen and pancreas. It is thus used in treating infection and inflammation and for diabetes. It is given in all diseases associated with weakness, debility and anemia.

Don sen strengthen the stomach and is used to treat hyperacidity and weak digestion.

Eleuthero   *Eleutherococcus senticosus*
                                           Araliaceae
PART USED: Roots and leaves
SYSTEMS AFFECTED: Heart, circulation, nerves and lungs
PROPERTIES: Cardiac tonic
          Antispasmodic

Eleuthero is a relative of ginseng that is used for its general tonic properties and for its calming effects. It is used in conditions for which ginseng would be considered too stimulating.

Eleuthero is considered by the Chinese to be the best medicine for treating insomnia. It is also extensively used for bronchitis and chronic lung ailments.

In the treatment and prevention of heart disease, eleuthero is used to lower blood pressure and reduce cholesterol levels. It has been used to treat arthritis, low blood oxygen, impotence and stress. It is a mild herb and must be used in large doses, about eight to thirty grams per day, depending upon the severity of the ailment. The leaves are stronger and are taken two to eight grams per day.

Ephedra   *Ephedra sinica*
                                                         Equisetaceae

PART USED: Stems and branches
SYSTEMS AFFECTED: Adrenals, lungs and heart
PROPERTIES: Stimulant
             Diaphoretic
             expectorant
             astringent

Ephedra is useful for asthma, bronchitis, coughs and other con-
gestive conditions. It should be used only for those with a Yang
constitution and are not deficient, as it is a strong stimulant that
would debilitate the adrenals of one who is already exhausted and low
in energy. It is good for colds and flus and for those fevers that are
without sweating. Ephedra increases blood pressure, and therefore
should not be used by people with hypertension.

There is also an American ephedra (desert tea), which is used similarly but is much milder.

Fu ling   *Poria cocos*
                                                         Polyporaceae

PART USED: Whole fungus
SYSTEMS AFFECTED: Kidneys
PROPERTIES: Diuretic
             Nervine
             expectorant

This fungus is considered one of the finest diuretics. It is used to
rid the body of excess moisture and the attendant emotional imbalances of insecurity, apprehension, fear and instability. It is used to
treat kidney weakness, lung congestion and insomnia. It helps to
expel and transform mucus.

It is nutritive and tonifying, helping the spleen, pancreas, stomach
and nerves. Thus it is prescribed in all wasting diseases. It is also used
for the treatment of hyperactivity in children.

Fu ling comes in both red and white colors. The red fu ling, called
muk sheng, is considered best for nervous, restless conditions.

Ginseng   *Panax ginseng*
                                                         Araliaceae

PART USED: Root
SYSTEMS AFFECTED: Heart and circulation; general effects on the
                  whole body

PROPERTIES: Alterative
               Cardiac tonic
               Hepatic tonic
               Stimulant

Ginseng is considered the king of all tonics. It provides a stimulation to the entire body energy to overcome stress and fatigue and to recover from weakness and deficiencies.

Ginseng has a very beneficial effect on the heart and circulation and is used to normalize blood pressure, reduce blood cholesterol and prevent atherosclerosis. It nourishes the blood and is thus used to treat anemia. By reducing blood sugar levels, it is useful in managing diabetes.

Ginseng is not used with any diseases where there is inflammation, burning sensations, high fever and other Yang conditions (see the "Diagnosis and Treatment" chapter). Ginseng is used for women with deficiency diseases, lowered resistance and lack of hormonal balance, but is not used with Yang conditions, such as excessive menstrual flow.

There are many grades of ginseng available. *Panax ginseng* comes from China and Korea, and is either dried (white), steamed and dried (which changes the color naturally to red) or extracted. I suggest using the red ginseng, the best being shiu chu roots from China.

Honeysuckle (Japanese)   *Lonicera japonica*
                                          Caprifoliaceae

PART USED: Flowers
SYSTEMS AFFECTED: Blood and liver
PROPERTIES: Alterative
               Antipyretic

Honeysuckle figures prominently in all Chinese detoxifying formulas. It is mostly used for all acute infectious and inflammatory conditions. It is very valuable for inflammatory skin diseases such as poison oak and various other rashes. It can be used alone or together with chrysanthemum flowers for treatment of acute flus, fevers and other similar conditions. It is not considered to be a medicine for chronic diseases and so is not intended for extended usage.

The infusion, prepared by steeping an ounce of the flowers in a pint of water, may also be applied externally for skin infections.

Ho shou wu   *Polygonum multiflorum*
(also known as Fo-Ti in the U.S.)   *Polygonaceae*

PART USED: Root
SYSTEMS AFFECTED: Kidneys, liver, blood, pancreas and spleen
PROPERTIES: Hepatic tonic
            Alterative
            Diuretic

Ho shou wu is a rejuvenating tonic that will restore energy, increase fertility and maintain strength and vigor for those who are advanced in years.

I recommend its use as a strengthener of the kidneys, liver and blood. It plays an important role in the treatment of all deficiency diseases. Ho shou wu is excellent for use in treating both hypoglycemia and diabetes.

The Chinese claim that it will keep the hair black, and benefit the muscles, tendons, ligaments and bones. Ho shou wu accomplishes this by preventing premature aging.

Licorice   *Glycyrrhiza glabra*
                                           Leguminosae

PART USED: Root
SYSTEMS AFFECTED: Lungs, stomach, intestines, spleen and liver;
                      general effects on the whole body
PROPERTIES: Expectorant
            Alterative
            Demulcent
            Laxative

Licorice contains substances similar to the adrenal cortical hormones. For this reason, it is very beneficial in treating adrenal insufficiency and other glandular problems. However, large and frequent doses will exacerbate hypertension.

Licorice can safely be added to tonics and detoxifying herbal formulas to alleviate the harsh stimulating aspects of bitter herbs without interfering with the beneficial aspects associated with their use. It is considered one of the most important herbs of Chinese medicine and is frequently prescribed as part of Chinese herbal formulas.

It is a proven remedy for all kinds of stomach and intestinal ulcers. It also has a stimulating action and helps counteract stress.

By itself, licorice is a good remedy for flu, colds, debility and all lung problems. It is a very good expectorant for treating coughs and bronchial congestion. For colds and flu, combine licorice with stimulating herbs, such as black pepper, sage, juniper, cayenne or ginger. Licorice root can be smoked for relief of sore throat and hoarseness.

Licorice is beneficial to the liver and for this it is often mixed with equal parts of peony root. It is a safe sweetener for diabetics. It is a good mild laxative that can be given to children and persons who are debilitated.

As a detoxifier of the blood, it can be combined favorably with echinacea, dandelion, red clover, burdock, sassafras or sarsaparilla.

Herbal pills can be made by decocting licorice with other herbs, straining and then slowly simmering down the liquid until a thick paste is formed. It is then rolled into little pills and dried at low heat or in the sun.

Lycii
Lycium chinenses
Solanaceae

PART USED: Berries
SYSTEMS AFFECTED: Blood, liver, kidneys and lungs
PROPERTIES: Nutrient tonic (Yin)
          Antipyretic
          Alterative

Lycii berries are a cooling tonic used to reduce fevers and thirst, and to treat bronchial inflammations. They aid in the removal of toxins from the blood by nourishing the liver and strengthening the kidneys. Lycii is often prescribed in the treatment of diabetes.

It is an ideal herb for meat eaters, as it is nourishing to the liver and kidneys like ginseng, but is a cooling, Yin tonic to balance the Yang effects of the meat.

Lycii is never used for acute fevers and colds because it is said to drive the fever deeper. It is best used for chronic, deficient, low-grade fevers with perspiration.

Pai shu
Atractylis lancea
Compositae

PART USED: Root
SYSTEMS AFFECTED: Kidneys, spleen, pancreas and stomach
PROPERTIES: Diuretic

Pai shu increases the energy of the body by eliminating excess moisture through a process that first eliminates excess sodium and other electrolytes. This process is effected without directly interfering with the kidney filtration process and thus as a diuretic, pai shu does not exhaust the kidneys as some other diuretics do. It is of very low toxicity and a major ingredient of the famous "Mu" tea blend. It is a tonic for the spleen and pancreas.

Pai shu is given for diarrhea, indigestion, edema, chest tightness, abdominal distension and vomiting.

It is often combined with other Chinese tonic herbs, such as those described in this chapter, to enhance their tonic properties.

Peony   *Paeonia albiflora*
                                            Ranunculaceae

PART USED: Root
SYSTEMS AFFECTED: Liver, blood, uterus and skin
PROPERTIES: Alterative
           Antispasmodic
           Hepatic tonic

Peony root is a liver tonic and is almost always used together with licorice root for treating all diseases stemming from an imbalanced liver function. It is also a good blood purifier, useful in treating skin eruptions and infections.

Peony is very useful in treating all female complaints, especially menstrual irregularity and abdominal pains associated with the menstrual cycle. It is nourishing to the blood and is used to treat anemia.

Rehmania   *Rehmania glutinosa*
                                            Scrophulariaceae

PART USED: Root
SYSTEMS AFFECTED: Blood, kidneys, bones and tendons
PROPERTIES: Cardiac tonic
           Diuretic
           Alterative
           Uterine tonic
           hemostatic

Rehmania is an important herb encountered frequently in Chinese herb formulas. It is used to purify and nourish the blood, strengthen the kidneys and heal the bones and tendons.

There are two forms commonly sold. One is the unprocessed root ("sang day"), which is considered the best for treating the kidneys and eliminating excess acids from the body. The other is a processed form ("sok day"), which is preferred for treating the blood. It is useful in treating anemia and heart weakness.

Rehmania is useful in helping build the body during recovery from illness, and it helps relieve fatigue. It is given to women to treat menstrual irregularities and infertility, as a tonic during pregnancy and to stop postpartum hemorrhage.

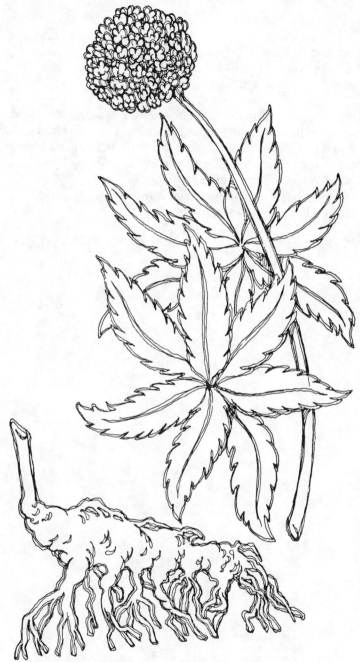

TIENCHI-GINSENG *(Panax notoginseng)*

*One of the best treatments for hemorrhage
and an excellent tonic for the heart.*

Tienchi   *Panax notoginseng*
                                         Araliaceae

PART USED: Root
SYSTEMS AFFECTED: Blood and heart
PROPERTIES: Hemostatic
            Cardiac tonic

Tienchi is one of the best treatments for hemorrhage. It may be applied directly to a wound or taken internally to stop bleeding (dose, three to nine grams). When cooked for about an hour in a tonic soup, it makes an excellent tonic for the heart, normalizing blood pressure and heart rate and improving circulation.

Tienchi is used to help maintain normal body weight, to prevent fatigue and to withstand stress.

10

OBTAINING AND STORING HERBS

In order for herbal remedies to be effective in the recommended doses, the herbs used must contain their full complement of active constituents. The potency of herbs depends on many factors:

1. the species;
2. the growing location and climatic conditions;
3. the time of harvest;
4. the method of drying and preserving;
5. the storage conditions;
6. the form of the herb;
7. the duration of storage.

Whether you harvest your own herbs or purchase herbs from a store, it will be of value to be familiar with all the factors that affect the potency of the herbs you use in healing.

SPECIES

In some cases, more than one species of plant will be sold under the same generic name. For example, "echinacea" is used to refer to both *Echinacea angustifolium* (Kansas snakeroot) and *Echinacea purpurea* (Missouri snakeroot). *Echinacea angustifolium* is probably more potent and is most commonly mentioned as the plant used in traditional native American medicine. Both have similar properties. However, *Echinacea purpurea* is more readily available and about one third the price of *Echinacea angustifolium*. Thus most herb stores will provide products made from *Echinacea purpurea*.

Similarly, "ephedra" may be used to describe *Ephedra sinensis* (ma huang or Chinese ephedra) or to refer to an American species of ephedra (desert tea or Mormon tea). But only the Chinese species contains large amounts of the active principle "ephedrin." In this case the availability and price in stores is similar, so that one or the other is likely to be carried.

In the case of ginseng, the term is properly used to describe both the Oriental ginseng, *Panax ginseng*, and the American variety, *Panax quinquefolium*. Both have similar properties, but the Chinese regard Oriental ginseng as warming and thus it is used as a winter tonic, while American ginseng is considered cooling and is used more as a summer tonic. An entirely different species, *Eleutherococcus senticosus*, which is a cousin of *Panax ginseng* with some similar properties, is often sold as "Siberian ginseng." Yet another plant, *Panax notoginseng*, is sold as "Tienchi ginseng." (See the chapter on "Herbs to Know" for further information on these species.).

There are two commonly used species of angelica, the Chinese variety, *Angelica sinensis* (dong quai) and the American and European species, *Angelica archangelica*. The Chinese variety is primarily used for its effects as a uterine tonic and antispasmodic, while the American species is used primarily for its warming, stimulant properties and in the treatment of lung diseases. The warming quality of the American species will help calm muscle spasms, and thus can partially match the antispasmodic properties of the Chinese species. However, the two are not equivalent in their effects and the Chinese species is superior as a treatment for all ailments of the female reproductive system.

Whenever there is any question as to the species of plant to use, it is best to investigate the matter more fully by consulting several sources of herbal information (see the Bibliography at the end of this book for some suggestions).

GROWING LOCATION AND CLIMATIC CONDITIONS

For any given species of plant, different growing conditions will affect the content of active principles. This will include the nutrient quality of the soil and the particular weather conditions during the plant's growth. In general, too little is known about how these factors influence the medicinal properties of the plant to allow much control in choosing the best quality.

For one who is following the principles of Simpling (see the chapter on "Theory of Using Herbs"), the local area is ideal. However, one should avoid picking herbs along heavily trafficked roads, since the exhausts from the vehicles will leave a residue on and in the plants.

When purchasing herbs from a store, one should realize that though many of the medicinal plants are available in the United States, the ones that are available commercially are often imported. This is because herb growing is a labor intensive enterprise and labor costs are too high in the United States compared to other countries, especially those of Eastern Europe, South and Central America. The major exception to this is the wildcrafting of herbs in the Appalachian region. Here, the poorer people can gather wild herbs in the surrounding forest area for a little extra income. The efforts of many individuals are revealed as a substantial quantity of herbs are brought to a central collecting area. These are then shipped around the country.

Herbs that survive a harsher climate are often believed to better help one through the harsher ailments.

TIME OF HARVEST

Herbs must be picked when they contain the highest amount of medicinal essences. This varies greatly throughout the year. The following are some general rules.

Leaves are picked just before the plant is about to begin flowering. At this time, the energy of the plant is focused in the upper portions. These and other plant parts should be picked after the morning dew has dried but before the hot sun has evaporated away the essential oils.

Flowers are picked just before they first reach full bloom. They will lose much of their value if picked later.

Berries and fruits are picked at the peak ripeness, as they are about to fall naturally from the plant.

When the aboveground portion of the plant is used, this usually refers to the combination of stems and leaves and is picked just before the plant begins to flower.

Barks and twigs of shrubs and trees are collected in the spring when the sap rises, when the leaves first appear.

Roots and rhizomes are collected in the fall, when the sap returns to the ground and as the leaves just begin to change color and the berries or seeds are mature. In some cases, such as sassafras, these are harvested in the early spring before the sap rises.

METHOD OF DRYING AND PRESERVING

Plant tops are gently washed, allowed to dry, then picked and hung in a well ventilated, dry, shaded area. Unless the whole plant is going to be used, the plant is hung upside down so that the sap will run from the stems into the leaves as it dries. They may be tied in small bunches, or they may be spread on a screen. If a screen is used, the plants should be turned each day to assure uniform drying.

Roots and barks are carefully scrubbed and then chopped before drying. The pieces should not be more than an inch thick after drying. Spread the pieces on a screen and turn daily. Those roots lacking volatile oils may be dried in direct sunlight, while the others should be dried in a warm shaded area.

A dryer that passes warm (about 100° F.) dry air upward through a series of screens can be used if air drying is not possible.

Drying will usually take three to four days. Most plants will lose half to three-quarters of their weight upon drying. They will generally retain about 10% of their weight as moisture.

Herbal properties may also be retained by other methods of preservation. Fresh herbs are used directly for making vinegar extracts (liniments), essential oils and salves (see "Methods of Application" chapter).

STORAGE CONDITIONS

Herbal properties are destroyed by heat, by bright light, by exposure to air, by the activity of plant enzymes and by bacteria and fungi. Enzyme activity and growth of microorganisms is promoted by heat and moisture. Volatile substances are readily lost to the air, and oxygen will destroy the properties of oils and other important substances in the herb.

Herbs should be kept in a cool, dry place with minimum exposure to air and sunlight. However, it is a mistake to hide herbs away in a dark closet or in dark jars if that will inhibit your use of them. It is much better to have them easily seen and readily accessible—they will not sit unused for long. Containers should be tightly capped. Clear plastic bags are almost useless, as they allow air to circulate and volatile substances are rapidly lost. Do not place herbs on a windowsill where they will have exposure to direct sunlight. Keep them at a safe distance from the kitchen stove and other sources of intense heat.

FORM OF THE HERB

When purchasing herbs, three forms are usually available: whole, cut/sifted and powdered. Whole herbs keep best, since air and microorganisms cannot get at the interior of the herb, but it is also more difficult to extract the essences. Whole herbs may be used for making tinctures, liniments and decoctions. Some herbs, such as small leaves and flowers, are usually available only in whole form or as powders. Herbs are cut and then sifted to remove powders for use in making teas. They are easy to strain when in this form and may also be used for most herbal applications, except for gelatin capsules and boluses. Powders do not keep as well because there is so much surface area exposed to air, moisture and light. Powdered herbs are specifically used for gelatin capsules, pills and boluses. It is often difficult to powder herbs finely enough for capsules, even with an electric coffee grinder, so it is advisable to purchase them already ground up. Powders may be used for most other applications, but they are more difficult to strain and must be separated through a cloth. An advantage to using powders is that they extract very quickly. Thus a tincture can be made in three days using powdered herbs but will require about fourteen days using whole herbs.

DURATION OF STORAGE

If herbs begin to lose their smell, taste and/or color they should be set aside for use in herbal baths for the body or for foot and hand baths. For this purpose, the older herbs can be mixed together indiscriminately. In general, one should restock one's herb collection every year or two. If herbs are purchased at a store, they have probably already been stored for one or two years since being harvested. These will then have a shelf life in the home of not more than one year. After that, they will have diminished potency. Herbs with aromatic oils will lose potency first, while heavy roots and barks and some seeds will maintain potency for considerably longer.

It is generally not necessary to keep a hundred herbs in stock. Rather, one should have a collection of about two dozen culinary herbs and spices regularly used in cooking, and about three dozen medicinal herbs, including those used most often and those that are more difficult to obtain. Then if other herbs are needed for treating a specific condition, one can purchase them at that time.

When making herb teas, it is often convenient to make a large batch, one quart to one gallon, and store it in a tightly closed bottle in the refrigerator. These teas will last for no more than about three days. When reheating, do not boil the tea. Tinctures and vinegar extracts, because of their antibacterial properties, will last for three years if stored in a cool place.

Oils, when stored with a minimum contact to air and kept in a cool place, will last for up to seven years. A small amount of Vitamin E added to the oil will greatly aid in preservation.

Salves and lotions may be preserved for several years by adding a small amount of tincture of benzoin. This is an important addition, since these may be applied to broken skin and thus must be kept relatively free of bacteria.

Poultices, boluses and fomentations should be made as needed and not stored at all.

11

MAKING AN HERBAL FORMULA

When using potent herbs, herbalists generally prefer using a mixture of several herbs according to a basic formula rather than using a single herb. This is because the single herb may have an effect that is too direct or too strong, or because a set of effects are desired that no single herb provides. One can think of the herbs as different colors. By mixing them together one can produce a tremendous variation in shades that aren't found in nature. The effects of the combination of herbs are different from the mere sum of the individual herbs going into the formulation.

An appropriately combined herbal formula is essential in the treatment of chronic ailments where many organ systems have been affected. The design of a tonic formula for a chronic ailment is a subtle art that must be developed with considerable experience. However, one may learn the way of herbs through the treatment of the acute ailments and thus gain experience to tackle the more difficult work with chronic problems.

For acute ailments, a general formula outline is:

1. use a large proportion (about 70–80% by weight) of one to three herbs that possess the primary property required to treat the ailment (expectorant for coughs, antibiotic and blood purifying properties for infections, warming properties for colds, etc.);
2. add a small amount of stimulant herb to promote the action of the primary medicine;
3. add a small amount of antispasmodic herb to reduce tensions in the body;
4. add a small amount of carminative or demulcent herb to provide gentle action and protection to the system.

The primary medicine makes up the major bulk of the herb formula and determines the basic action of the formula on the body. It is important that the secondary medicines—the stimulants, antispasmodics and demulcent/carminatives—not dilute the primary medicines. This is why about 70–80% of the herb formula is usually primary medicines.

Any herb may be a primary medicine, and the choice of the herbs to use will depend on the major symptoms of the body. Herbs always have a number of properties. By combining two or three herbs that share the property of greatest importance in treating the ailment, one will also get the other properties of these herbs. If the primary herbs are properly chosen, these additional properties will complement its action, providing other important effects that will assist in healing the body.

Of the secondary medicines, it is often the case that several essential properties can be found in a single herb, thus the formula may be simplified and the primary medicine will not be greatly diluted. Ginger, licorice, fennel seed, anise seed and cumin seed are examples of herbs that provide all three properties required of the secondary medicines. In some cases, however, specific herbs for each of the secondary properties will be desired. For example, if a strong demulcent is needed, an herb which is high in mucilage would be added.

The stimulant herbs have been discussed in the section on "Stimulation" in the "Herbal Therapies" chapter. A stimulant herb can be added to provide about 10% of the formula. Ginger root and cayenne pepper are two very commonly used herbs for this purpose.

Antispasmodics are important for two reasons. First, they relieve spasms directly associated with the ailment or as a result of tension/ nervousness in reaction to the disease symptoms. Second, they help prevent a reaction to strong effects of the primary medicine. Sometimes the bitter flavor of some herbs will upset one for a while, or the herbs will cause a slight nausea in the stomach. The antispasmodic relieves these reactions. Commonly used antispasmodics are lobelia, valerian and skullcap. Licorice is very useful for overcoming the strong bitter taste of some herbs. Antispasmodics make up about 10% of the formula.

Demulcent and carminative herbs soothe the system and counteract any irritating principles in the primary medicines. It is essential to use demulcents when giving diuretics, since if kidney stones are present, the diuretic may help release the stones, which would damage the tissues in the absence of a soothing demulcent. It is also necessary to use demulcents when using the more irritating diuretics (such as horsetail or juniper berries) and laxatives (such as cascara sagrada).

Carminatives are particularly useful to relax the stomach and intestines so that the herbal properties may be better assimilated. Demulcent herbs also help assimilation by softening the internal tissues, making them more absorbent. Demulcent/carminative herbs usually make up about 10% of the formula.

The treatment of chronic diseases requires a different approach. Because of the weakness developed during prolonged illness, one can't push the body too strongly in one direction. The herbs used must have a mild action and they must simultaneously strengthen all the affected systems. Since all herbs have a cleansing and eliminating effect, special care must be taken to use herbs whose eliminative power is mild.

I prepare a "signature formula" for the treatment of a chronic ailment, comprising a variety of herbs whose effects are matched to the particular condition of the person. All systems are affected to some degree. Because of the assortment of herbs with differing actions, I often add a small amount of licorice to balance the formula, harmonize the action of the herbs and avoid side effects. This practice has been successfully applied in China for many centuries. In fact, the Chinese refer to licorice as the "peacemaker."

A properly composed formula for the treatment of a chronic ailment should result in only gradual changes in the body's condition. If stronger symptoms of the disease arise after taking an herb tonic, the formula should be changed. As the chronic condition improves, the body becomes stronger and may eventually have the power to manifest the ailment as an acute disease (this process is called the "healing crisis"). At this time, it is possible to use stronger herbs with a more direct effect.

To maintain a mild character in a tonic herb formula, it is best to use complementary herbs. Hence if one uses a pungent or spicy herb, the irritating effects can be balanced by the use of a demulcent herb. When a diuretic or laxative is used, its effects can be toned down by adding an astringent. If anything in the formula is strong, it should be buffered by an appropriate complementary herb.

Just as one would use a mild action to treat chronic ailments because the energy is weak, one must generally avoid diluting the herbal formulas for acute diseases with many mild tonic herbs. In the acute disease, the individual is relatively strong and can best be helped to throw off the sickness by stimulating the natural defenses directly. A tonic may later be used to recover the full vitality of the body, which has been drained in the process of healing.

CHOOSING THE HERBS

Choosing herbs with the proper complement of effects is a relatively simple matter once the major properties of the important herbs are noted. Hence when a demulcent herb is to be used, marshmallow root is one of the best in a diuretic formula because it is also a diuretic; licorice is a demulcent preferred for tonics because it harmonizes the many herbs in that formula; slippery elm is used when extra nutrition is needed because of its high content of vitamins, minerals and carbohydrates. In choosing an antispasmodic, lobelia is used in treating acute ailments because of its strong direct action; valerian is used in more Yang tonics to treat superficial chronic ailments; skullcap is preferred to treat deeper and more debilitating chronic ailments affecting the nerves. Of the carminatives, cumin, fennel and anise seeds are very useful since they also have stimulant and antispasmodic properties, but they are without tonic value and are therefore used only in medicines for acute ailments. On the other hand, angelica is a carminitive with tonic properties, which may be successfully used in the treatment of chronic ailments.

A NOTE ON FOLLOWING THE RECIPES

The recipes that follow are designed for use with the herbal powders or the cut form of the herb. Proportions are given in parts by weight. When using a powder, let the powder settle to the bottom of the liquid extract and carefully pour off the clear extract for use. Alternatively, the liquid may be strained through a cheesecloth or paper filter. If the cut form is used, the extract is simply strained through a tea strainer. The advantage of powders is that they extract more fully and quickly than the cut form. They have the disadvantage of losing potency more quickly during storage and being more difficult to strain.

When whole herbs or seeds are used, they should first be crushed or bruised using a mortar and pestle. In making formulas that are to be capsuled, if the powder cannot be purchased, the herbs may be ground in an electric coffee and spice grinder. Pills can be made with a coarser powder. Alternatively, the formula may be used to make a tincture, in which one teaspoon (sixty drops) is taken in place of two gelatin capsules. (Note that dosages have assumed a body weight of about 150 pounds; people who weigh less will require a proportionately smaller dose.)

In some cases, the herb components of the formula have been divided into primary and secondary categories to demonstrate the use of this method of formulation. However, it is often the case that the primary and secondary properties are contained in the same herb and in these cases no division has been made. Some of the herbs contributing to the secondary properties (stimulant, antispasmodic, demulcent/carminative) have been indicated.

Herb recipes are given in parts by weight, so that the total amount of the formula to be made can be adjusted to your needs and the availability of the ingredients. As a simple guide, use one-half ounce of herb for a one part measurement. When taking the herbs for acute ailments, it is best to divide the daily dosage into smaller doses taken frequently throughout the day if it is convenient to do so. This way, the herbal properties will be continuously available for the body to use as needed.

Dr. Christopher's Lower Bowel Tonic

This is a very useful formula for treating all bowel problems. It will help to regulate bowel movements and restore tone to weakened bowels. This formula is also used in the treatment of hemorrhoids. Take two capsules, two or three times per day.

> *Primary:* Cascara sagrada—2 parts
> Bayberry bark—1 part
> Rhubarb root—1 part
> Goldenseal—1 part
> Raspberry leaves—1 part
> *Secondary:* Lobelia—1 part (antispasmodic)
> Ginger root—1 part (stimulant/carminative)

Combine together the powdered herbs and fill gelatin capsules, or add one part slippery elm and make small pills.

Antispasmodic Formula (acute medicine)

This is an all-purpose first aid remedy for a variety of emergencies, including shock, cramps, hysteria and poisonous bites and stings. It is also a good gargle to clear the voice, cut mucus and treat pyorrhea and sores in the mouth. Applied externally, it is used to treat pains and muscular spasms. Use fifteen drops in a half glass of hot water every hour or as needed for internal applications.

     Primary: Lobelia—1 part
                 Skullcap—1 part
                 Valerian—1 part
                 Myrrh gum—1 part
                 Black cohosh—1 part
 Secondary: Licorice—$\frac{1}{2}$ part (demulcent/harmonizer)
                 Ginger root—$\frac{1}{2}$ part (stimulant)

Steep the herbs in boiled water, one pint for six ounces of herbs, for one-half hour. Strain and add one pint apple cider vinegar.

Nerve Tonic (for chronic ailments)

Use this nerve tonic to treat chronic nervousness, muscular spasm or emotional instability. Take two teaspoons, three times a day.

          Black cohosh—1 part
          Hops—1 part
          Lady's slipper root—1 part
          Skullcap—1 part
          Lobelia—1 part
          Valerian—1 part
          Camomile—1 part
          Wood betony—1 part
          Hawthorn berry—1 part (demulcent)
          Ginger root—1 part (stimulant)

Mix the herbs thoroughly and use four ounces of herbs per pint of alcohol to make a tincture, Shake daily and allow to extract for two weeks. Then strain.

Sleep Formula

To achieve a sound sleep, drink this tea throughout the day, one-quarter cup three times, after meals, and one-quarter cup before going to bed.

   Primary and Hops—1 part
     secondary Valerian—1 part
      qualities Passion flower—1 part
    combined

Use one ounce of herbs steeped in a pint of boiled water for twenty minutes.

Female Corrective Tonic
(for women who have meat in the diet)

This tonic is used over an extended period of time to strengthen the genitourinary tract. Take two capsules or one teaspoon of tincture morning and night. After six weeks of use, go without using the formula for one week.

> Blessed thistle—1 part
> Cramp bark—1 part
> False unicorn root—1 part
> Squawvine—1 part
> Uva ursi—1 part
> Goldenseal—3 parts
> Ginger root—1 part (stimulant)
> Angelica or dong quai—1 part (antispasmodic)

Mix the powdered herbs and place in "00" capsules, or make a tincture using four ounces of herbs per pint of alcohol. Use with a half cup of raspberry leaf tea.

Female Corrective Tonic (for vegetarians or women who eat a low protein, high carbohydrate diet)

Of great benefit in correcting all menstrual irregularities.

> Dong quai—1 part
> Lovage—1 part
> Peony—1 part
> Rehmania—1 part
> Ginger root—$\frac{1}{2}$ part (stimulant)

Combine pieces of the herbs together in water (four and one-half ounces of herbs per quart) and cook slowly for forty-five minutes. Use as soup. The herbs may be cooked a second time.

Menstrual Cramps Formula

> *Primary:*   Cramp bark—1 part
>   Angelica or dong quai—1 part
>   Squawvine—1 part
> *Secondary:* Ginger root—$\frac{1}{2}$ part (stimulant)
>   Lobelia—$\frac{1}{2}$ part (antispasmodic)

Mix powdered herbs and fill "00" capsules. Take two or three as needed.

Composition Powder

This is a mixture of stimulant herbs that may be used for stimulant therapy (see the chapter on "Herbal Therapies") or to enhance the effects of other herbs. In the early stages of an acute disease, composition powder should be taken hourly.

Primary: Ginger root — 2 parts
Bayberry bark — 1 part
White pine — 1 part
Cloves — $\frac{1}{8}$ part
Cayenne — $\frac{1}{8}$ part
Secondary: Licorice — $\frac{1}{4}$ part (demulcent/harmonizer)

Steep one teaspoon of the combined powders in a cup of boiled water for fifteen minutes, covered. Drink the liquid poured off from the sediment.

Liver Tonic

This tonic helps rebuild the liver. It is useful in the recovery from hepatitis, liver sclerosis and toxicity from a bad diet.

Oregon grape root — 1 part
Wild yam root — 1 part
Dandelion root, raw — 1 part
Licorice — $\frac{1}{4}$ part (demulcent)

Simmer the herbs in distilled water (three ounces of herbs in one quart of water) for forty-five minutes. Refrigerate. Take two tablespoons, three or four times a day between meals. Do not add sweetening. If desired the licorice content may be slightly increased.

Bladder/Kidneys Tonic

This is a good tonic for the entire genitourinary tract and will serve as a good all-purpose diuretic. If you are ever in doubt as to what systems of the body are imbalanced, according to some practitioners of Chinese medicine it is generally best to treat the water element (bladder and kidneys). Take one-half cup of the tea four times a day, after meals and before going to bed.

Buchu — 1 part
Uva ursi — 1 part
Parsley root — 1 part
Cleavers — 1 part

Bladder/Kidneys Tonic — cont'd
                    Juniper berries — 1 part
                    Marshmallow root — 1 part (demulcent)
                    Ginger root — $\frac{1}{4}$ part (stimulant)
Combine the herbs and simmer one ounce of herbs in one pint of distilled water for twenty minutes.

Nerve Stimulant Formula

This is a powerful vitalizer for the entire nervous system; it is a general stimulant, and aids in digestion and elimination. Take three to four tablespoons, three or four times a day.
                    Prickly ash bark — 4 parts
                    Irish moss — 1 part (demulcent)
                    Bayberry bark — 1 part
Combine three ounces of herbs per quart of distilled water and let stand for two hours with occasional stirring. Then bring to a boil for thirty minutes and strain while hot. Add one cup of black molasses and one cup of glycerine to the strained liquid. Boil slowly for five minutes, stirring constantly. When it is cool, bottle and tightly cap.

Gallstone Formula

This formula will be helpful in reducing the symptoms of gallstone irritation and will aid in dissolving and removing the stones.
       Primary: Dandelion root — 1 part
                    Parsley root — 1 part
                    Lemon balm — 1 part
     Secondary: Ginger root — $\frac{1}{2}$ part (stimulant)
                    Licorice — $\frac{1}{2}$ part (demulcent/harmonizer)
Simmer the roots in water (two quarts water for every two ounces of herbs) for about an hour, reducing the volume by half through evaporation. Add the lemon balm and let steep for twenty minutes without additional heating. Strain and take one-half cup every two hours.

Liver and Kidneys Formula

This formula is used for treating acute ailments of the liver and kidneys.
       Primary: Juniper berries — 1 part
                    Dandelion root — 2 parts
     Secondary: Marshmallow root — $\frac{1}{2}$ part (demulcent)
                    Ginger root — $\frac{1}{2}$ part (stimulant)

Simmer the herbs for ten minutes (two quarts of water for every four ounces of herbs), then cool and strain. Take one-half cup, three times daily.

Internal Infections and Inflammations

Use this combination to treat serious internal infections.

    Primary: Echinacea—3 parts
Secondary: Marshmallow root—1 part (demulcent)
           Cayenne pepper—$\frac{1}{4}$ part (stimulant)

Fill "00" gelatin capsules with the combined herb powders and take two capsules every two hours.

Heartburn Formula

In this formula, the herbs each contain primary and secondary characteristics.

        Marshmallow root—6 parts (demulcent)
        Hawthorn berries—6 parts
        Peppermint—1 part (stimulant)

Simmer marshmallow root and hawthorn berries (one quart of water for every three ounces of herbs) for twenty minutes. Remove from heat and add the peppermint. Let steep ten minutes. Strain and drink one-half cup of tea every two hours.

Heart Tonic

Useful for treating high or low blood pressure or arhythmia. Take one teaspoon of the tincture with one tablespoon of wheat germ oil, three times daily.

        Hawthorn berries—6 parts
        Motherwort—3 parts
        Ginseng—3 parts
        Don sen—3 parts
        Ginger root—2 parts (stimulant/carminative)
        Comfrey root—2 parts (demulcent)

Combine four ounces of the herbs with a pint of alcohol (vodka, gin or brandy). Cap tightly and shake once or twice daily for fourteen days. Pour off the extract and strain out the herbs.

Children's Nervine

For hyperactive children and all nervous problems. Give three to seven drops of the tincture as needed.

>Camomile−2 parts
>Catnip−2 parts
>Valerian−2 parts
>Lady's slipper−1 part
>Hawthorn berries−1 part

Add four ounces of the herbs to a pint of brandy and extract for two weeks, shaking daily.

Prostate Tonic

This formula will dissolve kidney stones and clean out sediments and infection in the prostate.

>Gravel root−1 part
>Uva ursi−1 part
>Parsley root−1 part
>Goldenseal root−1 part
>Cayenne−1 part (stimulant)
>Juniper berries−1 part
>Marshmallow root−1 part (demulcent)
>Licorice−$\frac{1}{2}$ part (demulcent)

Mix together the powdered herbs and fill "00" gelatin capsules. Take two capsules, morning and night.

Glandular Balance Formula

This formula provides natural hormone-like substances.

>Licorice−1 part (demulcent)
>Black cohosh−1 part
>Sarsaparilla−1 part
>Dong quai−1 part
>Ginseng−1 part
>Kelp−1 part
>Goldenseal−$\frac{1}{2}$ part
>Ginger root−1 part (stimulant)
>Lobelia−$\frac{1}{2}$ part (antispasmodic)

Mix the herb powders and fill "00" capsules. Take two capsules, three times a day.

All-Purpose Liniment

Goldenseal — 1 part
Myrrh gum — 2 parts
Cayenne — ½ part

Mix herbs together in apple cider vinegar (three and one-half ounces of herbs per quart of vinegar) and cover tightly. Shake mixture once each day for seven days, then strain.

Eyewash

For red, tired or strained eyes, wash eyes twice a day.
Goldenseal — 1 part
Eyebright — 1 part
Bayberry bark — 1 part
Red raspberry leaves — 1 part

Mix herbs and make a tea, using one teaspoon of herbs in one-half pint of water. Allow to cool and keep refrigerated. Make fresh each week.

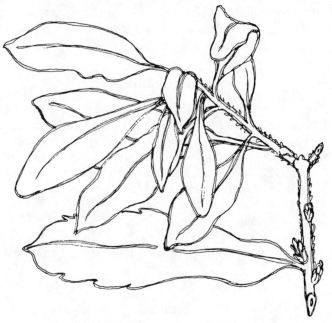

BAYBERRY (*Myrica cerifera*)

*Useful wherever an astringent is required, it is also
a stimulant that raises vitality and resistance to disease.*

Healing Salve

This salve is very useful in the treatment of all skin rashes, swellings, wounds and eruptions.

Calendula flowers — 1 part
Plantain leaves — $\frac{1}{2}$ part
Mugwort or wormwood — $\frac{1}{2}$ part
Comfrey leaves — $\frac{1}{2}$ part

Boil the herbs in lard or clarified butter (one pound of lard for every four ounces of herbs) over low heat until leaves are crisp. Strain and store in a wide-mouthed jar. The ointment can also be made with oil and beeswax (see the chapter on "Methods of Application").

Chickweed Salve

For the treatment of itching and rashes.

Fresh chickweed — 12 ounces
Vegetable shortening or oil — 16 ounces
Beeswax — 2 ounces

Melt the shortening and beeswax in a pan, then combine ingredients and place in the oven in a stone jar for about three hours; strain through a fine wire strainer while hot.

Comfrey Paste

This formula, provided by Dr. Christopher, can be used topically to heal burns, fractures, sprains and cuts. For third degree burns, wash the affected area thoroughly and apply with a bandage. Do not disturb for three days, thus allowing formation of new skin tissue to take place. The honey will keep the burn from getting infected.

Comfrey leaves or root — 3 parts
Lobelia — 1 part
Wheat germ oil — $\frac{1}{2}$ part
Honey — $\frac{1}{2}$ part

Combine herb powders with other ingredients and store in a wide-mouthed jar.

Poultice

This is used for drawing infections and in treating painful and swollen joints.

Plantain — 3 parts
Comfrey — 3 parts

Marshmallow root—1 part
Lobelia—1 part
Cayenne—⅛ part

Blend the herb powders together and add enough honey/wheat germ oil mixture (equal parts) to form a paste. Spread on gauze and apply over the affected area. Cover and leave on all day and night.

Bolus

This is used to draw out toxins and reduce cysts and tumors in the vagina or rectum. (See the chapter on "Methods of Application".)

Squawvine—1 part
Slippery elm—1 part
Yellow dock—1 part
Comfrey—1 part
Marshmallow root—1 part
Chickweed—1 part
Goldenseal root—1 part
Mullein leaves—1 part

Mix the powdered herbs together and add a tablespoon of the herbs to a small amount of melted cocoa butter to form a pie-dough consistency. Roll the mass to form the bolus. Refrigerate to solidify the cocoa butter and then allow to reach room temperature before applying.

Jeanne Rose's Spring Tonic

This valuable tonic is also used for treating acute ailments such as mumps, sore throats, indigestion, urethritis, abscessed teeth and infections of all types. Take two to four capsules twice daily.

Primary: Echinacea—2 parts
Yellow dock—1 part
Goldenseal—1 part
Ginseng—1 part
Secondary: Ginger—½ part (carminative/stimulant)

Combine together the powdered herbs and fill gelatin capsules, or make a tincture using four ounces of herb to a pint of alcohol, taking one-half to one teaspoon doses.

12

TREATMENTS FOR SPECIFIC AILMENTS

The suggestions in the following pages are typical types of treatments for specific ailments. On the basis of the information in preceding chapters, you can design alternative treatments to fit the particular nature of the ailment and to utilize those herbs and foods immediately available. Proportions are given in parts by weight.

In case you wish to make a formula but are lacking one or two ingredients, try to use a substitute with similar properties. If an ingredient were simply left out, the other ingredients would then be present in unusually high proportion and the effects might be somewhat different. When instructions are given to make a tea, it is also possible to make a tincture (see the chapter on "Methods of Application"), and when the instructions are given to fill gelatin capsules it is possible to use pills—or again one may simply use a tincture. The most consistent rule is to use common sense in determining the best method to apply the therapy. Remember to adjust the dose of internal medicines to the body weight of the person being treated (see the section on "Herbs for Children" in the "Cautionary Notes on Herb Use" chapter).

Continue to use the therapy for several days and follow the appropriate instructions on diet. Do not expect to get immediate changes in the condition after drinking a single cup of the tea, although in several cases this will occur.

Abscesses

Internal:
Prepare capsules of:
> Echinacea powder
> Chaparral powder

Alternate echinacea and chaparral, two capsules every two hours. After the infection subsides, reduce frequency of dose to every four hours.

External:
Make a poultice of:
> Plantain leaves—2–3 leaves, crushed
> Comfrey leaves—1–2 leaves, crushed
> Cayenne pepper—a pinch
> Marshmallow root powder—a pinch

Apply directly to affected area.

Note: This combined treatment is very effective for any type of infection, provided a balanced diet is strictly adhered to. It may be helpful to accompany this treatment with an herbal laxative or lower bowel tonic.

Acne and Skin Problems

Internal:
Use a good blood purifier, such as:
> Echinacea—2 parts
> Red clover—1 part
> Kelp—1 part
> Burdock—1 part
> Dandelion root—1 part
> Licorice—$\frac{1}{2}$ part

Fill gelatin capsules with the powder and take two capsules every two hours until the condition is greatly improved.

Or make a tea of:
> Sassafras—1 part
> Sarsaparilla—1 part
> Dandelion—1 part
> Burdock—1 part
> Licorice—$\frac{1}{2}$ part

Simmer one ounce of herbs in a pint of water for thirty minutes. Take one cup, three times daily.

External:
Use aromatic steam from:

> Elder flowers—2 parts
> Eucalyptus leaves—1 part

Use one ounce of herbs in a pint of boiled water in a bowl. Cover the head with a cloth and lean over the bowl to get the full benefit of the aromatic steam for five minutes.

Note: Skin eruptions are often caused by dietary imbalance, either by consuming too much meat, white sugar, denatured flours, eggs and stimulants (including spices) or by lack of wholesome foods such as whole grains, fresh vegetables, fruits and balanced protein. Skin ailments will often follow or accompany ailments of the lung or colon.

Arthritis and Rheumatism

Internal:
Use a good blood purifier, such as:

> Oregon grape root—6 parts
> Prince's pine or parsley root—6 parts
> Sassafras—3 parts
> Prickly ash bark—3 parts
> Black cohosh—3 parts
> Guaiacum—3 parts
> Ginger root—2 parts

Make a tea using one ounce of herbs to a pint of water, simmered for thirty minutes. Add a small amount of senna if necessary to regulate the bowels. Take one-half cup of the hot tea every two hours to induce perspiration. Between doses, take a nerve tonic tincture or powder with warm water. A simple combination of equal parts skullcap, valerian and lady's slipper will prove useful. Take two capsules or one teaspoon of the tincture.

External:
Apply warming herbs to promote circulation. Make a poultice, fomentation or liniment using:

> Ginger root—2 parts
> Cayenne—1 part
> Lobelia—$\frac{1}{2}$ part

Note: The intake of animal foods, alcohol, sugar and denatured foods should be reduced as these promote the deposit of uric acids in the joints. Avoid dampness and coldness of the joints, and use rubefacients or circulation-promoting herbs externally.

Back Pain

Internal:

Use a diuretic tea, such as:

> Juniper berries — 1 part
> Uva ursi — 1 part
> Parsley root — 1 part
> Marshmallow root — 1 part

Simmer two ounces of the herbs in two pints of water for fifteen minutes in a tightly covered pan. Strain and take one-half cup, three to four times daily.

Or use a diuretic, antispasmodic combination, such as:

> Prince's pine — 6 parts
> Valerian — 1 part
> Lobelia — 1 part
> Ginger root — 1 part
> Marshmallow root — 1 part

Simmer two ounces of the herbs in two pints of water for thirty minutes and take one cup three times a day or more often until relief is obtained.

In cases where there is inflammation, try:

> Echinacea — 4 parts
> Lady's slipper — 1 part

Make a tincture and take five to ten drops every two hours.

External:

Apply as a fomentation *equal* parts of:

> Comfrey root
> Horsetail
> Gravel root
> Marshmallow root
> Lobelia
> Ginger root

Simmer one ounce of the herbs in a pint of water for thirty minutes. Dip red flannel or a piece of thick cotton cloth into the solution and apply or wear to bed as warm as possible each night, using a plastic sheet to protect the bed from dampness.

Note: When there is back pain it is often symptomatic of deeper organic defects. Most back pain originates from kidney and bladder weakness. Various toxins otherwise eliminated through the kidney and bladder urine are deposited in surrounding tissue areas, especially the spinal joints of the lumbar region. If the back pain is accompanied by inflammation, it is often the case that nerves will become irritated, resulting in shooting pains called sciatica.

Burns

Internal:
Make a tea of:

> Comfrey leaf—2 parts
> Red clover blossoms—1 part
> Nettles—1 part
> Skullcap—1 part
> Marshmallow—1 part

Use one ounce of herbs per pint of water. Drink one-half cup every two hours, along with two capsules of equal parts echinacea and comfrey root powders.

External:
Apply immediately the gel pressed from aloe vera leaves. Make a poultice of calendula mixed with comfrey mucilage (see "Comfrey" in the "Herbs to Know" chapter) and a pinch of lobelia. For pain, add a pinch of echinacea or kava kava powder.

Coldness and Cramps

Internal:
Make a winter tonic using:

> Cramp bark—2 parts
> Angelica root—2 parts
> Squawvine—2 parts
> Raspberry leaves—2 parts
> Camomile—1 part
> Ginger root—1 part
> Lobelia—1 part

Add about six ounces of this combination to a quart of good quality dry wine. Heat gently in a covered container, but do not boil. Let stand for a day, then strain and bottle for use. Take one tablespoon three times daily, twenty minutes before meals.

External:
Apply a fomentation of ginger root.

Note: Avoid eating cold and watery foods. This formula is useful for the treatment of coldness, negative emotional states, deficiency, irregular menstruation and menstrual cramps. It will also be useful for all muscular cramps.

Colds, Flus, Fevers and Upper Respiratory Diseases

Internal:
If the ailment is due to overeating, use of alcohol, exposure to wet, damp, cold or excessive activity, use sweating therapy. For this a tea is made with *equal* parts of:

        Elder flowers
        Peppermint

Catnip, yarrow or lemon balm tea may be used instead. Take one or more cups of the infusion and follow immediately with a hot bath. Then go to bed with several covers to provoke perspiration. Use regular doses (every four hours) of one teaspoon garlic oil and two capsules of composition powder (see the chapter on "Making an Herbal Formula"). In case of fever make a tea of sweet basil with a pinch of black pepper. If the disease is caused by blocked food in the stomach, a lobelia emetic might be beneficial (see the "Herbal Therapies" chapter) to clear the stomach through vomiting.

If the ailment is accompanied by weakness, emaciation, paleness, low fever, clear or white discharge or is occurring in a person who has a deficient diet, low in protein, use a tea of *equal* parts:

        Dandelion root
        Burdock root
        Angelica root
        Chicory root
        Elecampane

Take one-half cup of the decoction every two hours. After the acute stage has passed, take one or two capsules of ginseng root a day to help overcome the deficient condition and build the body's defenses.

External:
Apply a rubbing oil of eucalyptus oil or a commercial combination such as Tiger Balm. For coughs, see the section on "Coughs and Sore Throats" in this chapter.

Note: Before treating a cold, flu or fever, determine whether the disease is due primarily to excess (Yang condition) or deficiency (Yin condition) as described in the chapter on "Diagnosis and Treatment." Those with a Yang condition should use a warm liquid diet and sweating therapy, while those with the Yin condition should avoid cold foods and should rely on teas, broths, mucousy grains, steamed vegetables, seaweeds and chicken soup. A Chinese tonic soup is of great benefit for treating the deficient condition (see the section on "Tonification" in the "Herbal Therapies" chapter and the section on "Chinese Herbs" in the "Herbs to Know" chapter).

Constipation and Diarrhea

Internal:
For a good remedy for either diarrhea or constipation take:

> Rhubarb root — 6 parts
> Slippery elm — 1 part
> Cinnamon — 1 part

Add enough water to make a mucilage from the combined powders and form little pea-sized pills. Dry with low heat, and then dip them in a little melted beeswax. Take two to seven pills, three times a day. The beeswax covering allows the pill to enter the small intestines before releasing its properties. One of the best formulas for all bowel complaints is Dr. Christopher's lower bowel tonic (see the chapter on "Making an Herbal Formula"). Use two capsules three times daily — the amount may be increased if results are not adequate. For constipation, one may also use a bulk laxative made by mixing:

> Psyllium seed
> Flax seed
> Chia seed

Use in any combination, soaking two to three tablespoons overnight in a cup of tea made from equal amounts of licorice and raisins. Take three tablespoons at a time, each hour.

For diarrhea and dysentery, make a tea of blackberry root bark (see the "Herbs to Know" chapter) and take one-half cup every two hours until the condition is relieved.

Note: Diarrhea is another form of constipation where the underlying cause is failure to assimilate food properly. The use of whole grains, bran and a balance of a few fruits and vegetables will help eliminate this problem, provided harmful denatured foods are removed from the diet. For children or persons who are weakened, a mild laxative is a tea of licorice and raisins or a tablespoon of sesame or olive oil taken in the evening.

Coughs and Sore Throats

Internal:
Make a cough syrup using *equal* parts:

> Elecampane
> Wild cherry bark
> Licorice
> Comfrey root
> Coltsfoot
> Lobelia

Cook down the decoction until a syrupy consistency is achieved (see the section on "Syrups" in the "Methods of Application" chapter). Take a tablespoon every hour or as needed.

Fill gelatin capsules with the powders of *equal* parts:

>Slippery elm
>Bayberry bark
>Comfrey root
>Mullein

Take two capsules every two hours along with one teaspoon of garlic oil and five to ten drops tincture of echinacea. An enema using white oak bark tea is also helpful.

Note: Coughs and sore throats are often benefited by a short fast or a diet using warm vegetable broth and soupy grains.

Cramps and Spasms

Internal:

For a tea that is warming and antispasmodic, use:

>Ginger root – 1 part
>Cramp bark – 2 parts

Take as needed. Or use the tincture of lobelia, five to fifteen drops, the antispasmodic formula (see the chapter on "Making an Herbal Formula") or a tea of equal parts camomile and ginger.

External:

Use a ginger compress or heating oils such as camphor, wintergreen or Tiger Balm.

Note: Cramps are often caused by cold, thus one should keep warm and take warm foods and drinks. Usually it is better to abstain from solid food for a while. Calcium is an important mineral nutrient in the prevention of cramps.

Fevers with Sweating

Internal:

For fevers accompanied by excessive sweating, make a tea using:

>Cinnamon – 2 parts
>Peony root – 2 parts
>Ginger root – 2 parts
>Licorice – 1 part

Simmer one ounce of the herbs in a quart of water along with four dates for twenty minutes. Take three or four cups a day, and one-half hour after taking the tea, eat a small bowl of watery brown rice.

External:
Make a tofu plaster by squeezing out the water from tofu and then mashing it together with 20% pastry flour and 5% grated fresh ginger root. Apply directly to the skin.

Headaches

Internal:
Make a tea of *equal* parts:
> Skullcap
> Valerian
> Rosemary
> Camomile
> Peppermint

Take one-half cup of the decoction (prepared in a tightly covered pot) every hour.

External:
Apply a stimulating oil to the forehead and temples, such as ginger, peppermint, wintergreen, Tiger Balm or Essential Balm (the latter two being commercial preparations from China).

Note: Headaches are usually caused by bowel and stomach disorders, or may be due to tension, stress, weak kidneys or sluggish liver function. The bowels and digestion should be regulated, perhaps with the use of a laxative such as a lower bowel tonic

Hemorrhoids

Internal:
Prepare a tea with:
> Dandelion root—2 parts
> Chicory root—1 part
> Cascara sagrada—1 part
> Oregon grape root—1 part
> Licorice—$\frac{1}{2}$ part

Using one ounce of herbs to one pint of water, make a decoction. Take one-half cup of the tea, two or three times a day.

External:
Combine:

>Witch hazel leaves—2 parts
>Bayberry bark—1 part
>Goldenseal—1 part

Make a strong tea using one ounce of herbs per pint of water. Add a pint of glycerine, and insert a small amount directly into the rectum with a dropper three times daily. Or make boluses and apply frequently (see the "Methods of Application" chapter). Also, see "Stoneroot" (in the chapter on "Herbs to Know").

Note: Hemorrhoids are often caused by sluggish liver function or liver obstruction. Hence the use of liver tonics are recommended. Another major cause of hemorrhoids is constipation. This is best corrected by balancing the diet and insuring that sufficient fiber is taken. The hemorrhoids are shrunk by the application of astringent herbs. Goldenseal is also applied, as it is beneficial for the inflamed mucous membrane surface of the rectum.

Hoarseness of Voice

Internal:
Use equal parts of powdered:

>Licorice
>Calamus

Mix with a little honey and take one teaspoon, three to four times daily.

Warm the body with a tea made from:

>Sage—4 parts
>Fresh ginger—4 parts
>Black pepper—a pinch
>Cinnamon—$\frac{1}{2}$ part
>Cardamom—$\frac{1}{2}$ part
>Licorice—$\frac{1}{2}$ part

Simmer two ounces of the mixture in a quart of water in a glass or enamel pot for twenty minutes. Add a little milk and continue to heat for ten minutes. Flavor with honey if desired. Add garlic, ginger and black pepper to cooked foods.

Note: One should avoid cold foods, fried foods and sour-tasting foods (such as yogurt and citrus). Gargling with salt water is beneficial, using one teaspoon salt to a glass of warm water.

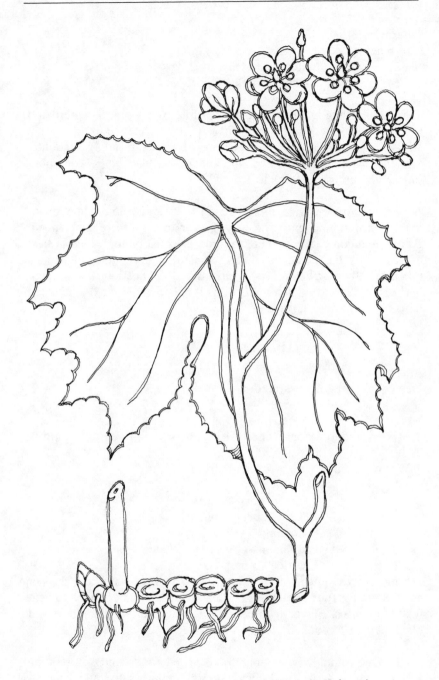

OREGON GRAPE ROOT (*Berberis aquifolium*)

*An aid to digestion and purification of the blood,
it is a tonic for all the glands.*

Indigestion

Internal:
Make an extract in any white wine using:

        Dandelion root—1 part
        Calamus root—1 part
        Gentian—1 part
        Angelica—1 part
        Valerian—1 part
        Ginger root—$\frac{1}{2}$ part

Use two ounces of herbs to one pint of wine and let extract for two weeks. Take one tablespoon before and after meals.

Infections and Blood Poisoning

Internal:
Mix the powders of *equal* parts:

        Echinacea
        Garlic
        Chaparral

Fill "00" capsules with the mixture. Take two every hour. As the symptoms subside, the dosage should diminish to three times a day for two weeks after all symptoms have disappeared.

External:
Make a poultice of:

        Plantain—2 parts
        Lobelia—1 part
        Marshmallow—1 part
        Cayenne—$\frac{1}{8}$ part

Insomnia

Internal:
Make an infusion using *equal* parts:

        Camomile
        Valerian
        Skullcap
        Catnip
        Wood betony
        Spearmint

Use one ounce of herbs per pint of water. Let steep ten minutes and drink before going to bed.

For incredible dreams and for nights when you can't allow sufficient time for sleep, make an infusion of:

> Kava kava—4 parts
> Alfalfa—1 part
> Spearmint—1 part
> Raspberry leaves—1 part
> Lemon balm—1 part

Vary the strength according to your needs, and sweeten with honey. The kava kava will produce a numbing effect on the tongue.

External:
Stuff a small pillow with hops and mugwort, and sleep on or next to it. Before bed, take a bath using herbs that are antispasmodic, nervine and/or sedative.

Note: Reduce the intake of strong stimulants, especially coffee and black tea, and normalize the daily schedule of meals and activities.

Kidney and Bladder Infections

Internal:
Make a tea of *equal* parts:

> Plantain
> Parsley root
> Marshmallow root

Take one-half cup every two hours. Also alternately take two capsules of echinacea or two capsules of chaparral along with the tea.

External:
Apply a hot ginger fomentation over the lower abdomen.

Note: The treatment should include a fast of one to three days, taking only warm vegetable broth and the herbs mentioned above.

Kidney Stones

Internal:
Make a decoction of:

> Gravel root—2 parts
> Parsley root—2 parts
> Marshmallow root—2 parts
> Lobelia—$\frac{1}{2}$ part
> Ginger root—$\frac{1}{2}$ part

Simmer two ounces of herbs per quart of water for about an hour until the liquid is reduced by half. Add an equal volume of vegetable glycerine to preserve. Take one-half cup, three times daily. Alternatively, one may make a tincture of the above herbs and take fifteen drops, three times daily.

Kidney Weakness

Internal:
A valuable Chinese formula is:

> Ginseng—3 parts
> Rehmania (unprocessed)—3 parts
> Fu ling—2 parts
> Licorice—1 part
> Ginger root—1 part

Make a decoction, using one ounce of the herbs for one pint of water. Take one-half cup, three times daily for three days.

A Western herbal formula is:

> Dandelion root—4 parts
> Parsley root—4 parts
> Marshmallow root—2 parts
> Ginger root—1 part

Simmer one ounce of the herbs in a pint of water for thirty minutes. Take one cup, three times daily. (See also "Buchu" and "Uva ursi" in the "Herbs to Know" chapter.)

Note: I would say that about 90% of the people in America suffer from weakened kidneys due to our dietary habits. This formula is thus useful for almost everyone.

Leukorrhea (White Vaginal Discharge)

Internal:
Make a decoction of *equal* parts:

> Uva ursi
> Parsley root
> Dandelion root
> Burdock root

Use one ounce of herbs per pint of water. Also, alternately take two capsules of equal parts echinacea, goldenseal and myrrh every two hours along with one half cup of the tea.

External:
Once a day use a douche made with white oak bark or bayberry bark tea.

Note: The treatment should begin with a one to three day fast, unless weakness or severe deficiency is present. Follow the fast with a light nourishing diet of whole grains, steamed vegetables and a small amount of beans and seaweeds.

Liver Ailments and Indigestion

Internal:
Mix *equal* parts of the powdered herbs:

> Calamus
> Wild cherry bark
> Gentian
> Oregon grape root
> Cascara bark
> Goldenseal
> Dandelion root
> Wild yam root
> Lobelia
> Ginger root
> Licorice

Fill "00" capsules. Take two capsules three times a day, with one cup of dandelion root tea, one-half hour before meals to improve digestion or after meals to influence the liver and stimulate the secretion of bile.

Note: This formula is good for cirrhosis of the liver, scrofula, indigestion, gas and constipation.

Menstrual Cramps and Irregularity

Internal:
Combine *equal* parts of:

> Dong quai
> Peony root
> Rehmania
> Licorice

Either make a tea by simmering one ounce of the herbs in a pint of water or use the powders in gelatin capsules. Take one-half cup of the tea or two gelatin capsules three times daily. This is a good tonic for regulating the menstrual cycle and reducing cramping.

For painful menstruation, one can also make a tea of:

> Angelica root—1 part
> Cramp bark—1 part

Camomile — 1 part
Ginger root — ¼ part

Steep one ounce of the herbs in a pint of water. Take one-half cup of the tea, two or three times a day regularly.

Another valuable formula is:

Squawvine — 4 parts
Cramp bark — 2 parts
Wild yam root — 1 part
False unicorn root — 1 part

Simmer one ounce of the herbs in a pint of water for twenty minutes. Strain and take two to three tablespoons, three times a day.

Note: Avoid exposure to cold (eating cold foods, swimming or bathing in cold water) around the time of the menstrual period. Make sure there is adequate calcium in the diet.

Mucous Congestion

Internal:
Combine the powders of:

Black pepper — 1 part
Ginger root — 1 part
Anise seed — 2 parts

Add a little honey to form a paste-like consistency. Take one-half teaspoon, three times a day before meals.

Note: This is an Ayurvedic anti-mucus formula called "trikatu." It acts as a natural antihistamine, and it can be added to other herbal formulas whenever this action is needed.

Nausea

Internal:
Mix together the powders of:

Cinnamon — 3 parts
Cardamom — 1 part
Nutmeg — 1 part
Cloves — 1 part

Use one-quarter to one-half teaspoon in a cup of boiling water, steeped covered for ten minutes. Strain, and drink one cup every four hours or as needed. It can also be added to scalded milk with a little honey.

Nervous Diseases

Internal:
As an all-purpose nerve tonic, blend together *equal* parts:

         Lady's slipper
         Valerian
         Wood betony
         Skullcap
         Spearmint
         Lemon balm

Use the powders to fill gelatin capsules and take two, three times a day, or steep two tablespoons in a cup of boiling water for ten minutes, adding honey to taste. Drink one cup, two or three times per day.

For treating hysteria, withdrawal from alcohol and drugs (delirium tremens—the "D.T.'s") and insomnia, make a tea of *equal* parts:

         Lady's slipper
         Skullcap

Simmer in a closed pot for twenty minutes, strain and add honey to taste. Take one-quarter cup every hour, tapering off as symptoms subside.

To promote memory and mental clarity, use:

         Gota kola—3 parts
         Calamus root—1 part

Heat an ounce of the mixture in a half pound of clarified butter (ghee) for fourty-five minutes. Strain and store for use. Dosage is one teaspoon in a cup of warm milk with a little honey (if desired), taken twice a day.

Note: Nervous debility comes from a combination of lack of balance in diet, recreation, exercise and rest. The herbs will help speed recovery as these important factors are brought into better balance.

Poison Oak and Poison Ivy

Internal:
Use a blood purifying combination, such as:

            Chaparral—1 part
            Yellow dock—2 parts
            Echinacea—2 parts

Combine the powders in gelatin capsules, and take two capsules every two hours.

Calm the itching and reaction to the pain using antispasmodics, such as:

> Raspberry leaves—2 parts
> Kava kava—1 part
> Black cohosh—1 part
> Lobelia—½ part

Combine the powders in gelatin capsules and take two capsules, three times a day.

Make a detoxifying tea using Chinese chrysanthemum and honey-suckle flowers in roughly equal portions.

External:
Apply a poultice of:

> Comfrey root
> Marshmallow root
> Slippery elm
> Aloe vera
> Witch hazel

Use roughly equal parts of each. Or use mugwort, plantain and comfrey leaf.

Prostatitis

Internal:
Make a decoction of:

> Gravel root—1 part
> Uva ursi—1 part
> Echinacea—1 part
> Parsley root—1 part
> Ginger root—¼ part
> Lobelia—¼ part

Use one ounce of the herbs per pint of water and drink three or four cups of this tea daily until relief is obtained.

Note: This formula will help the blood and kidneys, which in turn will be of benefit in relieving problems of the prostate gland. (See also the prostate tonic described in the chapter on "Making an Herbal Formula.")

Stomach Acidity

Internal:
As a decoction or in gelatin capsules, use:

> Dandelion root—1 part

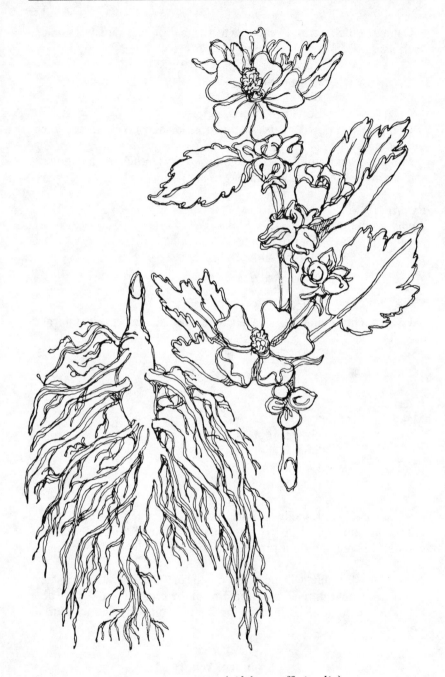

MARSHMALLOW (*Althea officinalis*)

The best source of vegetable mucilage.
Useful in all kidney and bladder formulas.

Stomach Acidity — cont'd

> Slippery elm — 1 part
> Goldenseal — $\frac{1}{8}$ part
> Calamus root — $\frac{1}{8}$ part

Take one-half cup of the tea or two gelatin capsules of the powder · every hour or as needed. Alternatively, combining a pinch of several kitchen spices, to total one teaspoon, in a glass of water will be very effective (see the "Medicines in the Spice Rack" section of the "Kitchen Medicines" chapter).

Note: Stomach acidity is due to imbalanced diet and must be controlled in the long run by becoming more in tune with the digestability of the foods being eaten.

Ulcers

Internal:

Combine *equal* parts of the powders of:

> Slippery elm bark
> Licorice
> Comfrey root
> Marshmallow root

Fill "00" gelatin capsules. Take two capsules, three or four times daily, especially before meals.

Note: The condition is treated by balancing the diet and using less meat and more vegetable protein, as is found in a combination of whole grains and beans. The bowels can be regulated with lower bowel tonic if necessary.

Vaginitis

Internal:

Combine powders of:

> Echinacea — 1 part
> Goldenseal — 1 part
> Chaparral — 1 part
> Squawvine — 1 part

Fill gelatin capsules. Take two capsules, three times a day, before meals. Also, take a teaspoon of garlic oil with meals.

External:

Make a tea of equal parts:

> Goldenseal
> Chaparral

Vaginitus—cont'd

> Comfrey root
> Kava kava

Use an ounce of herb per pint of water, and simmer gently for thirty minutes. Strain, cool and add one tablespoon vinegar per pint. Use as a douche once per day for one to three days.

Note: See also the section on "Leukorrhea" in this chapter.

Weakness

Internal:
Simmer in an open pot:

> Alfalfa—8 parts
> Comfrey root—2 parts
> Burdock root—2 parts
> Ginseng—1 part
> Dong quai—1 part

Use four ounces of herbs per quart of water. Cook this mixture for about one hour and strain. Return the liquid to the pot and add equal amounts of honey and barley malt syrup, totaling the same as the amount of herbal extract, so that the volume of the whole is doubled. Continue to heat and stir for five minutes to blend the ingredients. Take two tablespoons, three or four times a day, especially before meals.

A valuable Chinese formula is:

> Astragalus—6 parts
> Ginseng—3 parts
> Dong quai—3 parts
> Licorice—1 part

Simmer one ounce of herbs per quart of water in a nonmetallic container down to a pint. Take one cup of the tea, two to three times a day for three days.

Note: These formulas can be used as a good tonic for thinness, emaciation and general weakness.

Weight Reducing

Internal:
Combine the powders of:

> Kelp—5 parts
> Cascara bark—1 part
> Senna leaf—1 part

Cinnamon — 1 part
Licorice — 1 part
Poke root — 1 part

Fill "00" capsules with the mixture and take one or two capsules three times daily, before meals, with a cup of tea made of *equal* parts:

Chickweed
Cleavers
Fennel

Make an infusion with one ounce of herbs in a pint of water. This combination will have laxative, diuretic and balancing functions.

13

CAUTIONARY NOTES ON HERB USE

When properly used, herbs are the safest and surest medicines available. However, one must be well aware of the power of herbs both to heal and, if misused, to cause imbalance. Herbs produce no side effects when used in the amounts required to effect a cure. Negative effects occur only when one fails to observe the cautions that herbalists have recognized after many years of experience.

ESSENTIAL OILS

All essential oils are very concentrated substances that are irritating in large doses. Externally, one should avoid contact with the eyes, nose, mouth and all mucous membranes. Many of the essential oils are rubefacients intended to cause a mild irritation reaction to stimulate circulation in the area. If applied to the skin in large amounts they may cause a burning irritation.

Internally, essential oils are used only a drop or a few drops at a time, diluted in a cup of tea. In larger amounts they may cause severe toxic reactions. Recently, a fatal poisoning occurred from the ingestion of an ounce of pennyroyal oil. On the other hand, teas made from the herbs that yield these oils, and the use of small amounts of the oil as directed, cause no toxic reactions.

EMETICS AND LAXATIVES

Some herbs cause fairly strong reactions, and these are intended as part of the therapy. Thus emetics are meant to cause vomiting and laxatives are meant to cause strong bowel movements (strong laxatives are called cathartics or purgatives). The force of this reaction will depend upon the amount of herb taken. When these responses are expected, there is no problem, but the use of strong laxatives, such as senna leaf and cascara bark, will provide a very uncomfortable condition for anyone ignoring these properties. Many of the strong, bitter-tasting herbs will act as emetics if taken in large enough doses.

It must be remembered that emetics and laxatives, while stimulating the elimination of wastes, will also reduce the body's energy. Thus they should not be used by one who is already weak, nor should they be used repeatedly over an extended period of time.

When used in very small doses, emetic and laxative herbs will not cause noticeable eliminative responses, but they may reveal other properties. The most important example of this is lobelia, which is a strong emetic, most commonly used in small doses to act as an antispasmodic.

CUMULATIVE EFFECTS

Most herbs can be safely used in small quantities over a long period of time, but there are some that provide cumulative effects, which will be harmful if the herb is taken regularly without a break. These include goldenseal, which will affect blood pressure and digestion if taken continuously, and kava kava, which contains a substance that will be stored in the liver, and which taken in regular large doses may cause skin eruptions. Horsetail taken regularly may irritate the kidneys and cause some toxic reactions. These herbs should be used with adequate resting periods after any treatment lasting more than six days.

EXCESSIVE DOSES

Mild herbs can be taken in large quantities, and this is the practice in the art of Simpling. But more potent herbs will cause toxic reactions in large quantities. These include: poke, lobelia, goldenseal, horsetail, black cohosh, blue cohosh, aconite, mandrake and many of the very bitter-tasting herbs. With some herbs, such as black cohosh, you will be aware of taking more than a therapeutically useful dose by feeling nausea. The dose needs to be decreased. Sometimes, however, a mild nausea will be felt as a reaction to the bitter taste. The addition of a little licorice or ginger will often act to counteract this reaction.

SENSORY EFFECTS

Lobelia may cause a feeling of scratchiness at the back of the throat when taken in teas and tinctures. Both kava kava and cloves will cause a numbing effect on the tongue. Strong astringents, such as bayberry bark and myrrh, will cause a tightening sensation within the mouth when taken in teas and tinctures. Strong laxatives, known as purgatives, may cause intestinal cramping (called griping), and this is usually counteracted by using specific herbs (as mentioned, for example, in the chapter on "Herbs to Know"). Cayenne pepper will cause a very warm feeling in the stomach, and may also cause a burning sensation during defecation. Prickly ask bark will cause a strong sensation of heat in the stomach and may produce profuse perspiration.

TANNINS

Most herbs contain tannins, substances that bind up proteins and in so doing provide the property of being astringent. There appears to be a correlation between extensive drinking of tannin-rich teas and the occurrence of esophageal and stomach cancer. It is believed that the repeated effect of the tannins on the throat and stomach, especially in combination with other agents in the diet, may result in the formation of cancerous cells. In those countries where black tea *(Camellia sinensis)* is consumed in large quantities, the rate of esophageal cancer tends to be high. However, where the black tea is commonly taken with milk, the elevated cancer rate is not seen. This is because the tannins are rendered insoluble by the milk, the proteins of the milk being bound to the tannin.

One should use astringent teas as needed, but avoid excessive use. When an astringent herb is being used for properties other than astringency, a little milk should be added to neutralize the tannins. There is no reason to fear the occasional use of astringents internally or externally.

Herbs that are particularly high in tannins are the barks, such as bayberry, cascara and blackberry; some of the roots, such as yellow dock, sarsaparilla and comfrey; and a few leaf herbs, such as peppermint, uva ursi and cleavers.

FDA EVALUATION OF HERBS

The Food and Drug Administration has surveyed some of the available literature on chemical composition and pharmacology of herbs and has suggested that some herbs, commonly used as herbal medicines, are "unsafe." However, it must be realized that these herbs were not judged unsafe on the basis of proper usage, but only based on the presence of a known toxic substance or on the report of severe overdose reaction. Virtually all foods and medicines contain substances that are toxic in large enough doses, so this does not shed much light on the true toxicity of the herb. Among the herbs listed that are also mentioned in this book are calamus, lily of the valley, lobelia and mandrake.

In addition, by extracting ingredients from some herbs and feeding very large doses to laboratory animals, tumors have been induced in these animals. These substances are very weak carcinogenic agents and there is no evidence that the use of the herb itself is at all a health threat. Among the herbs which have been shown to contain a weak carcinogen are sassafras, nutmeg, cloves, basil and tarragon.

PREGNANCY

Pregnant women should carefully avoid using herbs that are emmenagogues. Oxytocic agents, which promote delivery, should only be taken during the last month of pregnancy. In general, strong uterine tonics such as dong quai and false unicorn are also not taken during pregnancy, except as directed.

Strong herbs and any kind of substance that has a strong effect on the body should be used with great care as they will also affect the developing fetus. Whenever possible, local applications, such as fomentations, liniments and salves, should be used in place of internal medicines.

HIGH BLOOD PRESSURE

Persons with a history of very high blood pressure should avoid herbs that stimulate the heart action or constrict the blood vessels. These include goldenseal, ginseng, licorice, lily of the valley and ephedra. Such persons should generally use only small amounts of stimulating substances and should use more of the antispasmodic, nervine and sedative herbs. However, two stimulants, cayenne pepper and garlic, also seem to be useful for reducing blood pressure.

CAUTION WITH HANDLING HERBS

When handling large amounts of poke root, for example when harvesting the roots, gloves must be worn because the roots contain substances that can pass through the skin and are toxic in large amounts. Nettles must also be picked with gloves, as the sting is very painful. Yellow dock applied to the area will be an antidote for nettles sting.

Cascara sagrada must be dried and stored for about one year before it is usable. Before this time it is too toxic. Blue cohosh powder must be handled with care as it is extremely irritating to the mucous membranes. Similarly, one must be careful handling cayenne powder.

Some herbs may cause allergic reactions; a couple of common examples are mugwort and orris root.

Aloe vera should only be taken internally in combination with ginger root, because alone it might cause cramping of the bowels.

HERBS FOR CHILDREN

When giving herbal remedies to children, the dosage should be decreased. As a general rule, the dose should follow the body weight, so that a forty pound child would get no more than half the dose of an eighty pound child. The doses recommended in this book are the adult doses, representing a body weight of about 150 pounds for purposes of calculation. *Therefore women weighing less than 150 pounds, for example, should begin with a lower dosage.* When treating very young children, only the very mild herbs should be used, such as lemon balm and catnip.

GATHERING WILD HERBS

Though it is a rare occurrence, it is possible to mistakenly identify herbs found in the wild, substituting a toxic plant for a healing herb. Always be sure of the identification of the plant species before gathering and using quantities of an herb. Recently, an elderly couple picked a plant they thought to be comfrey. They made a tea of this herb and were fatally poisoned. They had consumed a toxic dose of foxglove, a potent heart stimulant that is the source of digitalis. It is easy—and wise—to learn to distinguish foxglove and comfrey, but these people had not taken the time to become familiar with even the obvious botanical characteristics.

PESTICIDES AND CHEMICALS

Most of the herbs from the Appalachian region of the United States are collected from the forests, so these are completely natural products. However, the majority of other herbs are grown in large fields in foreign countries. The growers often use pesticides in producing these herb crops, so there may be some minor residues associated with these herbs.

When herbs are imported from certain tropical countries, they are fumigated with chemicals that destroy insects and their eggs when they arrive at United States ports. This is done in order to prevent exotic insects from entering the country.

A few herb manufacturers in the United States sterilize the herbs to destroy bacteria and fungi. It is not uncommon for dried herbs to contain thirty million bacteria per ounce! These are harmless bacteria, though they will contribute to the deterioration of the herb in the presence of excess moisture. The standard for drugs in the United States is to have not more than about one million bacteria per ounce. Those manufacturers attempting to match this standard will sterilize practically every herb. This is done by applying ethylene oxide gas. There are some minor residues thus left in these herbs.

Through consumer awareness of these practices, it may be possible to effect a shift away from the use of chemicals with a return to more natural methods of control, as has been done with organic produce.

DIAGNOSIS AND TREATMENT

This book provides basic principles for the diagnosis and treatment of a wide variety of ailments. These techniques are of particular value in treating minor acute ailments, curing long-term chronic ailments for which modern medicine is usually ineffective and as an adjunct to other therapies.

Every culture in the world has as an integral part of its social structure a group of healers who have a special knowledge of health, disease and the treatments of common ailments. Whenever one's own knowledge and experience of personal health and well-being is inadequate for treating these ailments, it is important to consult a trained healer. The herbal remedies in this book can be self-applied, but whenever there is any uncertainty about the nature of the ailment or the efficacy of the cure, a trained professional should be consulted.

Today there are many practicing herbalists and many doctors open to the idea of using natural methods of healing, including herbs. Seek out these individuals in your area and go to them for consultation when this seems appropriate.

Very special care must be taken if strong herbal remedies are used in conjunction with modern pharmaceuticals, as there might be adverse effects of the combinations. In such cases a doctor familiar with the pharmaceuticals must be consulted.

APPENDIX 1

Traveler's First Aid

CONDITION TO TREAT	HERBAL PREPARATION TO CARRY	METHOD OF APPLICATION
SUNBURN	aloe vera gel (may be purchased or squeezed fresh from the leaf)	Apply thin layer over affected area, reapply frequently.
BLEEDING	tincture of amaranth or powder or tienchi	Apply directly to wound, and internally as needed.
INFECTED WOUNDS	salve of equal parts goldenseal, myrrh and calendula	Apply to affected area.
SORE MUSCLES	liniment of equal parts eucalyptus, bay and rosemary, with one-quarter part lobelia	Apply to affected area.
BITES, SNAKE AND INSECT	tincture of echinacea	Apply to bite; also take internally one teaspoon every two hours for venomous bites.
REPELLING INSECTS	oil of pennyroyal and citronella	Apply to exposed areas, avoid contact with mucous membranes.

Condition to Treat	Herbal Preparation to Carry	Method of Application
POISON OAK AND IVY	tincture made with equal parts witch hazel, mugwort, comfrey root, plantain and white oak bark	Apply to affected area.
DYSENTERY AND DIARRHEA	capsules of blackberry bark and capsules of equal parts goldenseal and chaparral	Take two of each, every four hours.
CONSTIPATION	capsules of equal parts cascara, licorice and psyllium seed	Take two capsules every four hours.
IRRITATIONS	powder of equal parts comfrey root, slippery elm and marshmallow	For external use, add a little water and apply to affected area. For internal irritations, fill gelatin capsules and take two every two hours.
HYPERACIDITY	pieces of calamus root	Chew a small piece.
COLDNESS	capsules of composition powder, angelica, cayenne or prickly ash bark	Take two capsules as needed, not to exceed eight per day.
TO INDUCE VOMITING	Ipecac	Take as directed.
MENSTRUAL CRAMPS AND MUSCLE CRAMPS	capsules of dong quai, cramp bark or black haw	Take two as needed, not to exceed eight per day.
HEADACHE	tincture of rosemary	Fifteen to thirty drops as needed, internally.
INSOMNIA	tincture of equal parts valerian and kava kava	Take one teaspoon as needed.
FATIGUE	capsules of equal parts ginseng and astragalus	Take two capsules as needed, not to exceed eight per day.

Condition to Treat	Herbal Preparation to Carry	Method of Application
RED EYES	goldenseal tea preserved with tincture of benzoin	Make fresh before each trip, apply a few drops as needed.
COLDS AND FLU	oil of garlic and capsules of cayenne	Take a teaspoon of garlic oil and two capsules of cayenne every four hours.
POOR DIGESTION	tincture of agrimony or gentian	Take one to two teaspoons before meals.

How to carry: Put tinctures, liniments and oils in small plastic containers with flip-up dropper spouts. Carry capsules in plastic, multicompartment containers like those used by fishermen to separate small items. Salves, gels and powders can be carried in small, tightly capped jars.

How much to carry: Bring at least one ounce of the tinctures and oils; at least two ounces of the salves, liniments and gels; and at least eight of each capsule for each remedy you think you may need.

Other things to bring: Bandages, empty gelatin capsules, cloth and a small scissors.

APPENDIX 2

Where to Buy Herbs

It is always best to prepare herbal medicines from herbs you have picked and dried yourself, but this is not always possible. Many valuable herbs can easily be grown in semi-shaded areas of the garden where many "fussier" flowers and vegetables will not be able to flourish. There will always be a need to obtain the more exotic herbs and spices from reputable commercial sources. There is much room for improvement in the process of gathering, preparing and merchandising herbs and herbal products for the general market. This is the most significant area where I find that Chinese herbs are superior to our common Western herbs. Their herbs are picked or cultivated and prepared with great care. The Chinese herb stores in the Chinatown sections of our big cities are a sheer delight to visit. There one can see how carefully the medicines are treated, where several grades of a single herb are available at markedly different prices. This practice is hardly ever seen in the other markets in this country.

Most of the herbs mentioned in this book, as well as hundreds of others, can be obtained at most natural food stores, health food outlets and herb specialty shops. These stores can order herbs they do not usually carry upon your request. In case a good source of herbs is not available nearby you can order herbs by mail. Here is a partial list of reputable dealers that can provide herbs by mail or can be visited if you are in the area: (Be prepared to pay a handling charge for orders under $50 from some sources).

Nature's Herb Company   Green Mountain Herbs
281 Ellis Street   P.O. Box 2369
San Francisco, California 94102   Boulder, Colorado 80306

Pure Planet Products
P.O. Box 675B
Tempe, Arizona 85281

Sweethardt Herbs
P.O. Box 12602
Austin, Texas 78711

Superior Trading Company
(Chinese Herbs)
837 Washington Street
San Francisco, California 94108

Herb-Pharm
P.O. Box 116
Williams, Oregon 97544

Scarborough Fair
710 South Street
Philadelphia, Pennsylvania 19147

San Francisco Herb Tea
and Spice Company
2226 Union Street
San Francisco, California 94123

Taylor's Garden, Inc.
(Live Herbs and Seeds)
1535 Lone Oak Road
Vista, California 92083

Applegate Herbals
P.O. Box 1465
Grants Pass, Oregon 97497

Herbally Yours, Inc.
P.O. Box 26
Changewater, New Jersey 07831

Herbal Holding Company
P.O. Box 5854
Sherman Oaks, California 91413

House of Hezekiah
4305 Main Street
Kansas City, Missouri 64111

Old Fashioned Herb Company
P.O. Box 1000
Springville, Utah 84663

Christopher Enterprises
(Original Dr. Christopher formulas)
P.O. Box 352
Provo, UT 84601

APPENDIX 3

East-West Master Course in Herbology by Michael Tierra N.D., C.A.

This home study course in the principles of herbology presents the theories and approaches of Western naturopathic, Chinese, Japanese, American Indian and East Indian traditional medicine. It covers topics on herbal nutrition, gathering, preparation, diagnoses, and hundreds of herbs from around the world. The course is suitable for both the professional health therapist and the interested layperson.

Lessons are sent out twice each month, and there are thirty-six lessons in all. Each lesson includes a number of questions to be answered and returned. These will be evaluated and sent back to the student along with the next lesson. A certificate of completion will be issued at the end of the course. Total cost for the entire course is $300.

For a sample lesson send $3 to:

East-West Master Herb Course
c/o Michael Tierra
Box 712
Santa Cruz, CA 95061

BIBLIOGRAPHY AND SUGGESTED READING

The most valuable encyclopedic guide to the herbs and their uses is:
> *A Modern Herbal* (two volumes) by M. Grieve (Dover Publications).

This two volume set is available in paperback and is recommended for everyone who is seriously interested in herbal medicine. It provides extensive descriptions of the plants, of their history of use and of the medicinal actions ascribed to them. The book contains good details of the dose to be used.

An advanced guide to herbal formulas is:
> *School of Natural Healing* by Dr. J. R. Christopher (Bi World Industries).

It is a useful guide to hundreds of herbs with descriptions of many methods of application for a very wide variety of ailments.

To identify plants in the field, most plant guides will be helpful, but a book devoted specifically to herbs is:
> *Herb Identifier and Handbook* by Ingrid Gabriel (Sterling Publishing).

This guide is arranged according to the common names of the plants.

For brief references to American medicinal plants, two useful guides are:
> *A Guide to Medicinal Plants of the United States* by Arnold and Connie Krochmal (Quadrangle Press) and
> *Goldenseal/Etc.* by Louise Veninga and Ben Zaricor (Ruka Publications).

These have descriptions of the plants, their growing range and their medicinal uses.

Excellent plant illustrations are available in two books:
> *Health Plants of the World* by Bianchini, Corbetta and Pistoia (Newsweek Books) and
> *American Medicinal Plants* by C. F. Millspaugh (Dover Publications).

Health Plants has exquisite color drawings of many useful herbs and Millspaugh has very detailed prints of American species. Millspaugh's book contains descriptions of the physiological effects of herb overdoses that were used in the development of homeopathic prescribing.

To make herbal cosmetics, there are two readily available works:
> *Jeanne Rose's Herbal Body Book* (Grosset and Dunlap) and
> *Kitchen Cosmetics* (Panjandrum/Aris Books), both by Jeanne Rose.

The same author has prepared a handy guide to many commonly available herbs:
> *Herbs and Things* by Jeanne Rose (Grosset and Dunlap).

There are brief descriptions of hundreds of herbs with a long list of herbal recipes both new and old.

A more complete paperback guide to herb use is:
> *The Herb Book* by John Lust (Bantam).

Here you will find over 600 pages of cross-referenced descriptions of the herbs, their uses and methods of preparing many different and valuable concoctions.

If you are interested in the herbal roots, an excellent guide is:
> *Roots* by Douglas B. Elliott (Chatham Press).

This book has beautiful drawings of the roots and descriptions useful for both collecting and using them.

For additional information on Chinese herbs and medicine a valuable guide is:
> *A Barefoot Doctor's Manual*, revised edition (Cloudburst Press).

This has much information about the Chinese therapies for various ailments and gives the uses of many herbs, including the proper dose and formulation.

An encyclopedic guide to Chinese herbs that shows the Chinese characters as well as line drawings is:
> *Chinese Herbs* by John D. Keys (Charles Tuttle Company).

The descriptions of herb use are very brief.

For details about ginseng, the most important of the Chinese herbs, two books are recommended:

> *Ginseng: The Myth and the Truth* by Joseph P. Hou (Wilshire Book Co.). and
>
> *The Ginseng Book* by Louise Veninga (Ruka Publications).

Dr. Hou's book has a very extensive review of the scientific literature and reviews both commercial and clinical aspects of ginseng.

There are many guides to American Indian uses of herbs according to the region of the country and these can usually be found in your local bookstore. A general guide is:

> *Indian Herbalogy of North America* by Alma R. Hutchens (Merco).

This book includes extensive descriptions of the use of hundreds of American herbs and also has information about the Russian use of these medicinal plants.

For a textbook approach to herb drugs, a very good resource is

> *Pharmacognosy* by Tyler, Brady and Robbers (Lea and Febiger).

This book tells about the herbs that enter commerce, their source, their active ingredients and their uses by the drug industry. It is now in its seventh revised edition, but each edition of the book is useful. The older editions have more herbal information.

Another textbook is:

> *Medical Botany* by Walter H. Lewis and P. F. Elvin-Lewis (J. Wiley & Sons).

This book is arranged according to the systems of the body and then the plants useful in treating ailments of those systems, arranged by plant family. It has a very extensive bibliography.

If you are interested in pursuing the scientific details of herbs, including chemical constituents and pharmaceutical testing, use:

> *Chemical Abstracts, 5-Year Cumulative Subject Index*

at your local university. Look up the herb of interest according to the Latin binomial (genus and species).

An extremely valuable guide to medicinal plants with a good share of detail and scientific rigor is:

> *Medicinal Plants of the Mountain West* by Michael Moore (Museum of New Mexico Press).

It includes little known herbal effects, exact dosages, active ingredients, potential hazards and detailed descriptions of the plants.

To pursue further the dietary suggestions made in the chapter "A Balanced Diet" see:

Healing Ourselves by Naboru Muramoto (Avon).

This book presents the Japanese interpretation of Yin/Yang theory in terms of diet and other aspects of lifestyle.

For a regular update on herbal information, subscribe to:

Well-Being Magazine, Barbara Salat and David Copperfield, editors.

This do-it-yourself journal for healthy living specializes in herbal topics. Subscribe by writing to Well-Being Circulation Dept., Suite 921, 41 East 42nd Street, New York, NY 10017.

INDEX

Page numbers in boldface type refer to major discussions of spices or herbs in the "Kitchen Medicines" or "Herbs to Know" chapters. Page numbers in italic type refer to illustrations. Page numbers in boldface italic type refer to actual formulas or treatments for specific ailments.

A

Abdominal distension, 130
Abdominal pains, 6, 8, 72
Abortions, 45, 108
Abscesses, 88, 109, 124, 153; *155*
Aches, 70, 72
Achillea millefolium. See Yarrow
Acne, 77, 107, 109, 114, *155–56*
Aconite (*Aconite fischeri*), 22, 54, 55, 122, **123**; toxicity of, 177
Acorus calamus. See Calamus
Acute ailments, 65, 67, 84, 92, 110, 122; diagnosis of, 53; formulas for, 140–42, 143, 147, 153
Adrenals, 126, 128
Agrimony (*Agrimonia eupatoria*), 22, 44, 48, **76**. 184
Alcohol, for preparing herbs, 34, 39
Alcohol withdrawal, 78, 115, 170
Aletris farinosa, 94
Alfalfa (*Medicago sativa*), 17, 22, 41, 42, 54, **76–77**; nutrients in, 60, 77; in treatments, 166, 174
Allergic reactions to herbs, 180
Allium sativum. See Garlic

Allspice (*Pimenta officinalis*), 68
Almond oil, 45
Aloe vera (*Aloe vera*), 21, 22, 41, 44, 48, **77**; caution about, 180; in treatments, 158, 171, 182
Alteratives, 40–41, 66, 68, 69, 72, 73, 76–83 passim, 87–89, 91–96 passim, 102, 103, 106–14 passim, 117, 120–30 passim. *See also* Blood purification
Althea officinalis. See Marshmallow
Amaranth (*Amaranthus* spp.), 22, **77–78**, 182
Amenorrhea. *See* Menstrual problems
Analgesic herbs, 41, 92, 99, 100, 109, 121, 123
Anemia, 76, 91, 106, 122, 124, 125, 127, 130
Angelica (*Angelica archangelica*), 22, 41, 42, 45, 46, **78**, 108; dong quai vs., 124–25, 135; in formulas, 143, 146, 159, 165, 168, 183
Angelica sinesis. See Dong quai
Anise (*Pimpinella anisum*), 22, 42, 44, 45, 46, 65, **66**; in formulas, 66, 87, 141, 143, 169
Antacids, 41. *See also* Stomach acidity
Antiabortives, 41, 94, 116

E

sinus infection   Pe Min Kan Wan
chinese licorice/grated ginger tea
echinacea/golden seal tincture

Weights and Measures

1 pound = 453 grams
1 ounce = 28.3 grams
16 ounces (dry) = 1 pound
1 quart = 2 pints
1 pint = 2 cups
1 cup = 16 ounces (fluid)
1 teaspoon = 60 drops
1 tablespoon = 3 teaspoons
1 fluid ounce = 2 tablespoons
1 cup = 16 tablespoons

Capsules and Powders

15.4 grains = 1 gram
1 gram = 1000 milligrams (mg)
contents 1 "00" capsule = about 650 mg = 10 grains (well packed)*
contents 1 "0" capsule = about 500 mg = 8 grains (well packed)
Two gelatin capsules = one teaspoon of the tincture
Two tablespoons tincture = one-half cup of tea

*1 teaspoon of powder will fill about two "00" capsules. Thus one ounce of powdered herb will fill 40 to 50 "00" capsules or 50 to 70 "0" capsules, depending on the type of herb, fineness of powder and tightness of packing.

HOW MUCH IS AN OUNCE OF HERBS?

It is not necessary to use precise amounts of the herbs because the herbs will vary in their potency and individuals will vary in need, so the amounts suggested are useful approximations. The best way to measure out ounces is with a simple pan balance scale. These can be purchased from scientific supply stores, and from some drugstores. Gram scales are very useful and can be obtained for under fifty dollars. Kitchen scales are available for under twenty dollars. If you purchase bulk herbs a few ounces at a time, it is easy to divide up the package into roughly equal piles of one ounce each, based on the amount weighed out at the store.